Concise Review

For The

PTCB Exam

Brian Tuschl, Pharm.D.

Christopher Ardoin, BSPharm

TPS Healthcare Solutions, LLC
Tech Prep Solutions
PO Box 1164
Spring, Texas 77383
(832) 489-0561
(281) 435-7671

This edition published by Dog Ear Publishing
4010 W. 86th Street, Ste H
Indianapolis, IN 46268
www.dogearpublishing.net

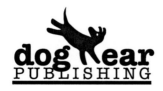

ISBN: 978-159858-261-1
Library of Congress Control Number:
This book is printed on acid-free paper.

Printed in the United States of America

Acknowledgments

We would like to express our appreciation and thanks to our families for their support while writing this book.

I would like to thank Jesus Christ; through Him anything is possible. I also thank my wife, Lyndi, who has been my rock and biggest supporter and also my children, Sarah, DeLanie and Gabriel, who have had much patience in the writing of this book. My gratitude and appreciation goes out to my parents, Marvin and Mona Tuschl, and my in-laws, Lannie and Lanez Scarborough, who are always very encouraging and supportive.

Many people have given their time and effort to help bring this book to completion. We gratefully acknowledge the assistance of the following:

Dana Kornreich, Pharm. D. Candidate
University of Houston College of Pharmacy
Houston, Texas

Arturo Martinez, Jr., CPhT
University of Houston
Houston, Texas

Duc Thang Nguyen, Pharm. D. Candidate
University of Houston College of Pharmacy
Houston, Texas

Ibukunoluwa I. Akindele, CPhT
University of Houston
Houston, Texas

Rebecca Forte, Pharm. D. Candidate
University of Houston College of Pharmacy
Houston, Texas

Carie Briggs, CPhT

Cheryl Bedenbaugh, M.S.

Kathryn Bao-Thu, Pharm. D.
University of Houston College of Pharmacy
Houston, Texas

Kenny Bedenbaugh

Alana McCarn, Pharm. D. Candidate
University of Houston College of Pharmacy
Houston, Texas

Lanez Scarborough, M.Ed

May Woo, RPh
University of Houston College of Pharmacy
Houston, Texas

LaTasha Wells, CPhT

Marvin Tuschl, Sr.

Eva Broussard, Pharm. D.

Cover, logo, and chapter designs by Arturo Martinez, Jr., Houston, Texas.

Table of Contents

Foreword

Raymond W. Hammond, Pharm.D., BCPS, FCCP

With the entry of the baby boomer generation into retirement age, there has been a vast increase in the need for pharmacies and pharmacy services. At the same time pharmacy education has increased to a minimum of a 6-year curriculum, resulting in the awarding of a doctorate degree and the profession has moved from a primarily dispensing profession to one that is more patient-oriented. Pharmacists of the 21st Century are assuming more responsibility in assuring that the patient's drug therapy is working, but not causing adverse effects. All of these factors have contributed to a shortage of pharmacists and an increased demand for pharmacists and pharmacy technicians. Societal, professional, and legal expectations make it necessary for the pharmacist to spend more time in direct patient care – medication therapy management, counseling patients on the proper way to take their medication and answering patient questions, monitoring the patient's response to therapy, and providing drug information and consulting services to physicians and other healthcare providers. For pharmacists to fulfill their patient care responsibilities, they must relinquish the major portion of their dispensing role to pharmacy technicians.

As pharmacy technicians assume a greater role in providing prescriptions to patients, state boards of pharmacy – in keeping with their role of protecting the public – are increasingly requiring that pharmacy technicians become certified. In many states, certification requires passing the Pharmacy Technician Certification Board Exam (PTCB). Most technicians prepare for this exam by completing a 2-year curriculum in a technical school, but such training is not currently a requirement for taking the PTCB Exam. Those without the resources and time to attend a technical school, or those looking for a "fast track" to certification, will find *Concise Review for the PTCB Exam* to be a useful tool in preparing for the exam.

Dr. Tuschl and Mr. Ardoin have prepared an excellent self-learning text that provides the essential information, practice problems, and self-assessment components to provide dedicated individuals with the knowledge and skills necessary to successfully pass the PTCB exam and attain pharmacy technician certification.

Introduction

This review guide is a valuable tool for individuals who are preparing to take the pharmacy technician certification exam. It is not intended to address all aspects of the pharmacy profession. Rather, its purpose is to teach quick study tips and the basic facts needed to pass the certification exam.

PTCB Exam Contents:
The exam consists of 100 multiple-choice questions. There will be 2 hours to complete the exam. A calculator may be used during the exam. The exam will cover the following topics:
1. Assisting the pharmacist (64%)
       a. brand and generic drug names
       b. drug usage
       c. drug side effects
       d. drug classes
2. Drug inventory control (25%)
3. Pharmacy administration and management (11%)

When taking the exam, remember to eliminate the choices that are obviously incorrect. This will narrow down the choices if having to guess at the correct answer. Only one answer will be correct. Make sure that each answer is read carefully before marking the final answer. Generally, it is not a good idea to go back and review the questions and make changes in the answers, if allowed. In most cases, the first selected answer is likely to be correct.

Helpful test-taking tips:
- Get a good night's sleep the night before the test.
- Bring a good watch for time keeping.
- Bring identification.
- Know the testing format.
- Read all possible answers before marking your choice.
- Eliminate incorrect answers when possible.
- Complete the entire test.

For more information, please visit the following websites:
- Pharmacy Technicain Certification Board- www.ptcb.org
- American Association of Pharmacy Technicians-www.pharmacytechnician.com

FEDERAL PHARMACY LAW

CHAPTER 1

PHARMACY LAW

1906 Federal Food and Drug Act
This act prohibits the sale of adulterated or mislabeled food, drinks and drugs.

1914 Harrison Narcotic Act
This act limits the transport of opium. In order to purchase opium, a prescription is required.

1938 Food Drug and Cosmetic Act
This act made the Food and Drug Act more comprehensive to include cosmetics. The act also defines misbranding or adulteration of drugs to be illegal.
- Requires drug companies to provide package inserts.
- Requires that a habit-forming drug to be labeled *"may be habit forming."*
- Requires that a new drug has to be <u>proven safe</u> under FDA guidelines before marketing.

1951 Durham Humphrey Amendment
This act distinguishes legend drugs (prescription) from over the counter drugs (OTC).
- Requires companies to label legend drugs *"**Caution: Federal law prohibits dispensing without a prescription.**"*
- Requires physician supervision for the purchase of legend drugs.
- Over the counter drugs without medical supervision are required to have on the label:
  - Product name
  - Name and address of manufacturer and/or distributor
  - Active ingredients
  - Quantities of all other ingredients whether active or not

1962 Kefauver-Harris Amendment
All drugs made from 1938 forward have to be proven <u>safe</u> and <u>effective</u>. This amendment was enacted due to birth defects caused by the drug **thalidomide** in Europe.
- Requires *"**Good Manufacturing Practices**"* GMP
- Stricter requirements are now placed on drug manufacturers seeking drug approval; manufacturers have to prove their drug to be safe and effective before marketing it.
- **FTC** (Federal Trade Commission), not the FDA, now handles drug advertisement.
- Requires that a **manufacturer must**:
  - Register annually
  - Report any adverse reactions
  - Be inspected every two years

1970 Comprehensive Drug Abuse Prevention and Control Act (Controlled Substance Act-CSA)
Drug Enforcement Agency (DEA) was formed which is a unit of the Justice Department. The controlled substances are now placed into schedules I–V which are based on abuse potential. Schedule I drugs have the highest potential for abuse and schedule V drugs have the least potential for abuse.

1970 Poison Prevention Packaging Act
This act requires <u>childproof packaging</u> on most drugs dispensed in a pharmacy. Drugs that are exempt from this act are drugs used in emergency situations, such as dispensing **nitroglycerin,** or if a drug is packaged in such a small quanity it would not harm a child under the age of five.

1983 Orphan Drug Act
This act enables the **FDA** to promote the research and marketing of drugs needed for the treatment of rare diseases. These drugs are made for such a small percentage of the population that the drug's demand does not make marketing and manufacturing in large quantities economically feasible.

1984 Drug Price Competition and Patent-Term Restoration Act (Hatch-Waxman Amendment)
This act streamlines the process for granting approval of generic drugs. It also gives manufacturers incentives to develop new drugs by giving patent extensions. This act allows generic drug companies the ability to rely on safety and efficacy findings of an innovator's drug after the expiration of the patent.

1988 Food and Drug Administration Act
This act established the FDA as an agency of the Department of Health and Human Services. Also, in 1988 the Prescription Drug Marketing Act was establised, which banned the sale, trade or purchase of drug samples. Any adverse drug reactions and outcomes should be **reported to the FDA.**

1990 Omnibus Budget Reconciliation Act (OBRA)
This act **requires** a pharmacist to <u>attempt or offer</u> to **counsel** patients on all new prescriptions. Pharmacists are now required to provide information on any drug being dispensed such as: name and description of the medication, and how much of the medication should be taken, side effects, contraindications, interactions, adverse effects of the medication, storage, refill information and what to do if a dose is missed.

1996 Health Insurance Portability and Accountability Act (HIPAA)
This act created rules and regulations regarding the privacy and security of patient health information (PHI-protected health information). This act provides limitations stating who can access, distribute and receive patient health information. It makes health insurance portable for employees switching jobs. It also includes provisions that make health care information more cost effective and efficient by requiring standardized electronic transmissions of claim information.

2006 Combat Methamphetamine Epidemic Act (CMEA)
This act limits the purchase of pseudoephedrine (pse) products to **3.6g of pse per day or 9g per 30 days.**

<u>Product Recalls</u>
When a pharmacy is notified of a drug recall, **lot numbers and expiration dates** are used to identify the affected drugs.
1. Class I recall:
> An <u>attempt</u> must be made **to notify the patient** that the drug he/she may be taking **could** cause **serious harm or death.**
2. Class II recall:
> The probability of serious harm is **not likely** and the effects may be temporary or reversible. This recall **does not go to the customer level** and is usually due to problems with consistency of potency.
3. Class III recall:
> Not likely to cause any serious adverse effects and **does not go to the customer level.**

OTC labeling must contain:
1) The name of the product, address of the manufacturer, packer, or distributor.
2) The net contents of the package.
3) The established name of **all** active ingredients and the quantity of certain other ingredients, whether active or not.
4) The name of any habit-forming drugs contained in the product, and any caution labels and warnings needed to protect the customer.
5) Adequate directions for use:
   a. Statements of the drug's intended conditions and purposes.
   b. It also must contain the normal dose used for a specific indication, the individuals age and their physical condition.
   c. The frequency and duration of administration and/or the application in relation to meals, onset of symptoms, or other time factors.
   d. The route, method or application of administration.
   e. What, if any, are the required preparations for use.

The Food, Drug and Cosmetic Act (FDCA) requires Prescription Labels to contain:
1) The name, address and phone number of the dispensing pharmacy.
2) The patient and doctor's name.
3) The prescription number and the date the prescription was filled.
4) The name of the drug, strength, quanity and the directions for use.
5) The name or initials of the dispensing pharmacist and/or technician.
6) Patient's address.
7) Expiration date, refill information and any precautions.
8) The statement "**Federal law prohibits dispensing without a prescription.**"
9) A package insert on selected drugs.

Package Inserts must contain:
1) Description of the drug.
2) Clinical Pharmacology.
3) Indications and usage.
4) Contraindications, precautions, warnings and adverse reactions.
5) Drug abuse, dependence and overdosage information.
6) Dosage, administration and how the drug is supplied.
7) The date of the most recent labeling revision.

Package inserts must be distributed with the following drug classes:
1) Oral contraceptives
2) Estrogen-containing and progestational drugs
3) Intrauterine contraceptive devices
4) Diethylstilbestrol products
5) Accutane
6) Metered-Dose inhalers

National Drug Code (NDC)
Each drug produced by a manufacturer is identified with a specific NDC number. The NDC number is composed of three sets of numbers, which identifies the manufacturer, drug, and pack size (e.g., 12345-6789-10).
1) The first **five** numbers identify the **manufacturer**. All drugs made by this manufacturer will have the same set of five numbers (e.g., all drugs made by manufacturer "X" will start with 12345).

2) The next **four** numbers identify a **specific drug** made by the manufacturer. Each drug will have its own number. If the manufacturer makes drug "X", then drug "X" will have its own specific middle four numbers (e.g., 6789). If the same manufacturer makes another drug, "Y", then drug "Y" will have the same first five numbers (12345) but a different set of middle four numbers (e.g., 7245).

3) The last **two** numbers identify the **package size.** For example, if a drug comes in a quantity of 100 tablets the last two digits may be 01 or if the drug comes in a quanity of 500 tablets the last two digits may be 05.

Schedule Drugs (Controlled Drug Substances-CDS)
Schedule I
- These drugs have <u>**NO**</u> accepted medicinal use in the United States.
- These drugs have the highest abuse potential.
  - Heroin
  - Peyote
  - LSD
  - Marijuana
  - Mescaline

Schedule II
- These drugs may **not** be refilled.
- The **ordering** of schedule II drugs requires a **DEA 222** form.
- The **returning** of out of date schedule II drugs requires a **DEA 222** form.
- These drugs have a high abuse potential that may lead to severe physical or psychological dependence.
  - Cocaine
  - Morphine
  - Amphetamines
  - Codeine
  - Opium
  - Methadone
  - Oxycodone
  - Hydromorphone
  - Fentanyl
  - Meperidine
  - Methylphenidate
  - Secobarbital

Schedule III
- These drugs may be refilled **5 times in a 6 month period.**
- These drugs have less potential for abuse or dependence than schedule I or schedule II drugs.
  - Vicodin (Hydrocodone/ Acetaminophen), Lortab, Lorcet, Norco
  - Tylenol No.3 (Codeine/ Acetaminophen)
  - Marinol (Drobabinol)
  - Anabolic steroids (Testosterone)
  - Cough syrups containing hydrocodone

Schedule IV
- These drugs may be refilled **5 times in a 6 month period.**
- These drugs have less potential for abuse or dependence than schedule II or III drugs.
  - Benzodiazepines (alprazolam, diazepam, lorazepam, etc.)
  - Phentermine
  - Pentazocine
  - Phenobarbital
  - Diethylpropion

Schedule V
- These drugs have less potential for abuse or dependence than schedule II, III, and IV drugs.
    - Antitussives with codeine
    - Antidiarrheals with opioid

*Schedule II-V drugs **must** have an auxiliary label that states *"Caution: Federal law prohibits the transfer of this drug to any person other than the patient for whom it was prescribed."*

Filing Schedule and Dangerous Drugs
A controlled substance inventory must be done at least once every 2 years, and the records must be kept for at least 2 years.
Prescription Filing Methods:
1) Two File System- Make one file for CDS CII-CV prescriptions provided that all **CIII-CV** prescriptions contain a **red "C" at least one inch high stamped on the lower right hand corner** of the prescription. There must be an additional file for all other prescriptions (non-controlled prescriptions).
2) Two File System- Make one file for CDS CII only. Make another file for all other prescriptions (non-controlled and CDS CIII-CV prescriptions) provided that the CIII-CV prescriptions contain a **red "C" at least one inch high stamped on the lower right hand corner** of the prescription.
3) Three File System- Make one file for CDS CII only, one file for CDS CIII-CV, and one file for all other prescriptions (non-controlled prescriptions).

Forms for Controlled Drug Substances
DEA 222
The DEA 222 form is used for the **purchasing** and **returning of outdated** CII drugs. The DEA 222 form comes in three copies:
1) **Blue copy:** the **purchaser** keeps the blue copy on file for at least two years. The pharmacy is usually the purchaser except when the pharmacy is sending back out-of-date drugs then it becomes the seller.
2) **Green copy:** The seller sends the green copy to the local DEA.
3) **Brown copy:** The seller keeps the brown copy on file.

DEA 106
The DEA 106 form is used to **report lost or stolen** controlled substances. A DEA 106 form is used when 5% of the yearly product sold is missing. For example, if 1000 tablets of vicodin are sold per year and one tablet is missing, legally, the pharmacist-in-charge (PIC) does not have to file a DEA 106 (the PIC can file a DEA 106, but it is not mandatory). If fifty or more tablets are missing (which would be 5% or greater of the total amount of vicodin sold within a year), then it is **mandatory** that the PIC report the missing drugs via the DEA 106 form.

DEA 41
The DEA 41 form is used to document the **destruction of controlled substances**.

DEA 224
The DEA 224 form is needed for a pharmacy to **dispense controlled substances**.

DEA 363
The DEA 363 form is needed to **operate a controlled substance treatment program** or **compound controlled substances**.

DEA 225
The DEA 225 form is needed to **manufacture** or **distribute** controlled substances.

Verifying the validity of a doctor's DEA number

A doctor that prescribes controlled medications **must** have a DEA number. This number consists of 2 letters followed by 7 numbers. The formula to verify the validity of a DEA number is the sum of the 1st, 3rd and 5th numbers added to twice the sum of the 2nd, 4th and 6th numbers. The total's last number should be the same as the last number of the doctor's DEA. This may sound a bit confusing, but as shown in the following example, it is really quite simple. Let's do it step by step.

For Example:
Dr. Hillman writes a prescription for Diazepam 5 mg, one every day, for a quantitiy of 30 tablets. The doctor's DEA is AH1264869. To verify the validity of the doctor Hillman's DEA follow these six steps.

Follow the six steps to verify Dr. Hillman's DEA
1) The first letter in the DEA number should be an A or a B.
2) The second letter should be the first letter of the physician's last name (Doctor Hillman's last name starts with an "H" so the second letter in the DEA should be an "H").
3) Now add the 1st, 3rd and 5th number, $1 + 6 + 8 = 15$.
4) Now add the 2nd, 4th, and 6th number and multiply by 2, $(2 + 4 + 6) \times 2 = (12) \times 2 = 24$.
5) Now add the two sums together, $15 + 24 = 39$
6) The last digit, 9, in the number 39 should match the last number in the DEA (AH1264869).

Practice problems
1) Which DEA number for Dr. Somebody is valid?
   a) BS1122681
   b) AS1236824
   c) BC1236547
   d) AS1465981

2) Which DEA number for Dr. Brown is valid?
   a) AB1654782
   b) BB8326452
   c) AB2364587
   d) AC1255478

Answers
1) a 2) b

Pharmacy Resources

Approved Drug Products with Therapeutic Equivalence Evaluations (Orange Book):
The Orange Book compares therapeutic equivalency of drugs using an alphabetical rating system. This book determines whether or not certain drugs may be substituted in place of others. 'A' rated products **can** be substituted because they are bioequivalent. 'B' rated products **cannot** be substituted because they are not bioequivalent. This book is **published yearly** and is also called FDA's approved drug products publication.

USP/NF US Pharmacopoeia/National Formulary:
USP/NF contains monographs and chemical characteristics of drugs. This book is published by a private organization.

USPDI US Pharmacopoeia Dispensing Information:
A three volume set:
> Volume I: Drug information written for a <u>health care provider</u>.
> Volume II: Drug information written for <u>patients</u>.
> Volume III: Therapeutic equivalency information and pharmacy law.

US Pharmacopoeia General Chapter 797:
This chapter states the procedures and requirements for pharmaceutical compounding of sterile preparations.

Drug Facts and Comparisons:
This book contains a comprehensive listing of drugs and comparative drugs. These drugs are organized by therapeutic class and provide general information with a list of monographs. There is also a listing of drug manufacturers, including addresses and phone numbers in the very back of the book. This book is **updated monthly**.

Drug Topics Red Book:
This book gives a listing of drugs by **pricing**, strengths, sizes, manufacturers, brands and generics.

Handbook on Injectable Drugs:
This book lists injectable drug information such as compatability, storage and dosages.

Physician's Desk Reference (PDR):
The PDR contains packet insert drug information intended for physicians and is published annually. It contains color pictures with a list of drug manufactures including their addresses and phone numbers.

Mosby's Complete Drug Reference:
Mosby's Drug Reference lists generic drugs in alphabetical order. It also contains additional drug information.

American Drug Index:
Drugs are listed alphabetically and provide brand, generic and the chemical names of the drugs. It gives a list of manufactuers, strengths and dosage forms of the drugs listed.

The Handbood of Injectable Drugs:
This book is used to determine the compatibility of medications that will be used in an IV bag. This reference shows the compatability, solubility and stability of medications.

Material Safety Data Sheets (MSDS):
MSDS provides information on **hazardous materials** that may be in the pharmacy and also provides information on disposal, storage, safe use and clean-up of these medications.

Pharmacy Law Questions

1. When ordering a CIII medication what document is required for proof of receipt?
   a. Blue copy DEA 222
   b. Green copy DEA 222
   c. Commercial invoice
   d. Drug report

2. Because federal and state record keeping requirements can vary in each state, which law should be followed?
   a. State law
   b. Federal law
   c. Most recent law
   d. Most stringent

3. For general laws concerning pharmacy rules and regulations, which law should be followed?
   a. State law
   b. Federal law
   c. Most stringent
   d. Least stringent

4. Which of the following is true regarding a doctor's DEA number?
   a. It is 7 digits in length
   b. A DEA number is necessary when filling a controlled drug substance
   c. The second letter of DEA is the initial of the doctor's last name
   d. All of the above

16

5. Which one of these DEA numbers for Dr. Wilson is correct?
   a. AW1287952
   b. BW4545698
   c. AW1437537
   d. AW1115424

6. Which statement is true regarding NDC numbers?
   a. The middle four numbers indicate a specific drug
   b. The 3rd set of numbers represent the manufacturer
   c. The NDC number can be found in Facts and Comparisons
   d. All the above

7. To whom are drug recalls, drug reactions and outcomes reported?
   a. DEA
   b. FDA
   c. JCAHO
   d. EPA

8. When drug manufacturers notify a pharmacy of a drug recall, how are the affected drugs identified?
   a. NDC number and manufacturer
   b. LOT number and expiration date
   c. Invoices
   d. None of the above

9. Which one of the following drugs would not require a patient package insert?
   a. Accutane
   b. Premarin
   c. Norethindrone
   d. Omeprazole

10. What do the first five, middle four and last two digits of an NDC number represent?
    a. Manufacturer, package size and drug
    b. Manufacturer, drug and package size
    c. Drug, package size and manufacturer
    d. Package size, drug and manufacturer

11. A list of drug package inserts could be located in which one of these books?
    a. Fact and comparison
    b. Drug topics
    c. Physician desk reference
    d. Merck index

12. What is the maximum amount of refills for CIII-CV prescriptions in a six month period?
    a. 10 refills
    b. 6 refills
    c. no refills
    d. 5 refills

13. Who may initiate the ordering of an investigational drug?
    a. Nurse
    b. Pharmacist
    c. Physician
    d. Hospital administrator

14. Who may order controlled drug substance schedule CI drugs?
    a. Physician
    b. Pharmacist
    c. Both
    d. Neither

15. The expiration date on a bottle of Naproxen is 8/08. When will this drug expire?
    a. The first day of August
    b. The last day of August
    c. The first day of September
    d. The last day of July

16. Which drug recall must go to the customer level?

    a. Class I
    b. Class II
    c. Class III
    d. Class IV

17. Which form is used to report lost or stolen drugs?

    a. DEA 222
    b. DEA 106
    c. DEA 225
    d. DEA 363

18. Which schedule has no legal medicinal use?

    a. Schedule I
    b. Schedule II
    c. Schedule III
    d. Schedule IV

19. Which drug does not require a childproof closure?

    a. Viagra
    b. Nitroglycerin
    c. Premarin
    d. Zyrtec

20. Which form is used when ordering CII drugs?

    a. DEA 106
    b. DEA 225
    c. DEA 222
    d. DEA 41

21. A prescription for Alprazolam may be refilled how many times?

    a. 0
    b. 1
    c. 5
    d. 6

22. If a doctor indicates 2 refills on a prescription for percocet 10mg, how may times may it be refilled?

    a. 0
    b. 1
    c. 2
    d. depends on the quantity written

23. What is the total number of tablets a customer will receive after using all of their refills on a prescription for vicodin #30 with 3 refills?

    a. 30
    b. 60
    c. 90
    d. 120

24. A prescription for Norco 10/325 mg with 2 refills is written and first filled on 1/1/2005, when will the prescription expire?

    a. 2/1/2005
    b. 4/1/2005
    c. 1/1/2006
    d. 7/1/2005

Law Answers

1.c 2.d 3.c 4.d 5.c 6.a 7.b 8.b 9.d 10.b 11.c 12.d 13.c 14.d 15.b 16.a 17.b 18.a 19.b 20.c 21.c 22.a 23.d 24.d

QUICK

DRUG

CLASSIFICATION

CHAPTER 2

DRUG CLASSIFICATION BY PREFIX OR SUFFIX

This table is an extremely important part of this book. In my teaching experience, students often get overwhelmed with the number of drugs in the pharmacy. At first glance, it seems impossible to learn all of the brand and generic drug names. This process can be made much easier by learning the prefixes and suffixes of common drugs dispensed. For example, if it is known that "statin" drugs are used to treat hyperlipidemia (high cholesterol), then it would be obvious that Simva**statin**, Prava**statin** and Lova**statin** are all drugs that can be given to lower cholesterol.

Quick Drug Classification by Prefix or Suffix				
Suffix or Prefix	**Drug Category**	**Class or Action**	**Brand**	**Generic**
-mycin	Antibiotic	Macrolides	Biaxin®, Biaxin XL®	clarithro**mycin**
			Ery-Tab®, E-mycin®	erythro**mycin**
			Ketek®	telithro**mycin**
			Zithromycin®, Zmax®	azithro**mycin**
-cycline	Antibiotic	Tetracyclines	Minocin®, Dynacin®	mino**cycline**
			Sumycin®	tetra**cycline**
			Vibramycin®, Adoxa®, Doryx®, Monodox®, Periostat®	doxy**cycline**
-floxacin	Antibiotic	Fluoroquinolones	Avelox®	moxi**floxacin**
			Cipro®	cipro**floxacin**
			Factive®	gemi**floxacin**
			Floxin®	o**floxacin**
			Levaquin®	levo**floxacin**
			Tequin®	gati**floxacin**
ceph-, cef-	Antibiotic	Cephalosporins	Ceclor®	**ceph**alor
			Cedax®	**cef**tibuten
			Ceftin®	**cef**uroxime
			Cefzil®	**cef**prozil
			Duricef®	**cef**adroxil
			Keflex®	**ceph**alexin
			Omnicef®	**cef**dinir
			Spectracef®	**cef**ditoren
			Suprax®	**cef**ixime
			Vantin®	**cef**podoxime
-cillin	Antibiotic	Penicillins	Amoxil®, Trimox®	amoxi**cillin**
			Dynapen®	dicloxa**cillin**
			Pen Vee K®, Veetids®	peni**cillin** V
			Principen®	ampi**cillin**
-cyclovir	Antiviral	Anti-Herpetics	Denavir®	pen**ciclovir**
			Famvir®	fam**ciclovir**
			Valcyte®	valgan**ciclovir**
			Valtrex®	vala**cyclovir**
			Zovirax®	a**cyclovir**

-pril	Antihypertensive	Angiotensin Converting Enzyme- Inhibitors (ACEI's)	Accupril®	quina*pril*
			Aceon®	perindo*pril*
			Altace®	rami*pril*
			Capoten®	capto*pril*
			Lotensin®	benaze*pril*
			Mavik®	trandola*pril*
			Monopril®	fosino*pril*
			Prinivil®, Zestril®	lisino*pril*
			Univasc®	moexi*pril*
			Vasotec®	enala*pril*
-sartan	Antihypertensive	Angiotensin II Receptor-Blockers (ARB's)	Atacand®	candes*artan*
			Avapro®	irbes*artan*
			Benicar®	olmes*artan*
			Cozaar®	los*artan*
			Diovan®	vals*artan*
			Micardis®	telmis*artan*
			Teveten®	epros*artan*
-osin	Antihypertensive, Benign Prostatic Hyperplasia (BPH)	α 1-Receptor Blockers	Cardura®	doxaz*osin*
			Flomax®	tamsul*osin*
			Hytrin®	teraz*osin*
			Minipress®	praz*osin*
			Uroxatral®	alfuz*osin*
-olol	Antihypertensive	Cardioselective β -Receptor Blockers	Kerlone®	betax*olol*
			Lopressor®	metopr*olol* tartrate
			Tenormin®	aten*olol*
			Toprol XL®	metopr*olol* succinate
			Zebeta®	bisopr*olol*
		Nonselective β -Receptor Blockers	Blocadren®	tim*olol*
			Inderal®	propran*olol*
			Corgard®	nad*olol*
		ISA (Intrinsic Sympathomimetic Activity)	Cartrol®	carte*olol*
			Levatol®	penbut*olol*
			Sectral®	acebut*olol*
			Visken®	pind*olol*
		Mixed α & β-Receptor Blockers	Coreg®	carvedi*lol*
			Trandate®, Normodyne®	labeta*lol*
-dipine	Antihypertensive	Calcium Channel Blockers (CCB's)	Adalat CC®, Procardia XL®	nife*dipine*
			Cardene®	nicar*dipine*
			DynaCirc®	isra*dipine*
			Norvasc®	amlo*dipine*
			Plendil®	felo*dipine*
			Sular®	nisol*dipine*

-statin	Antihyperlipidemia	HMG-CoA Reductase Inhibitors	Crestor®	rosuva*statin*
			Lescol®	fluva*statin*
			Lipitor®	atorva*statin*
			Mevacor®	lova*statin*
			Pravachol®	prava*statin*
			Zocor®	simva*statin*
-glitazone	Antidiabetic	Thiazolidinediones	Actos®	pio*glitazone*
			Avandia®	rosi*glitazone*
-glinide	Antidiabetic	Meglitinides	Prandin®	repa*glinide*
			Starlix®	nate*glinide*
-dronate	Osteoporosis	Bisphosphonates	Actonel®	rise*dronate*
			Boniva®	iban*dronate*
			Fosamax®	alen*dronate*
-tidine	Anti-ulcer	H2-Receptor Antagonists	Axid®	niza*tidine*
			Pepcid®	famo*tidine*
			Tagamet®	cime*tidine*
			Zantac®	rani*tidine*
-prazole	Anti-ulcer	Proton Pump Inhibitors (PPI's)	Aciphex®	rabe*prazole*
			Nexium®	esome*prazole*
			Prevacid®	lanso*prazole*
			Prilosec®	ome*prazole*
			Protonix®	panto*prazole*
-triptan	Anti-migraine	5-HT1 Receptor Antagonists (Triptan's)	Amerge®	nara*triptan*
			Axert®	almo*triptan*
			Frova®	frova*triptan*
			Imitrex®	suma*triptan*
			Maxalt®	riza*triptan*
			Relpax®	ele*triptan*
			Zomig®	zolmi*triptan*
-pam, -lam	Anti-anxiety/ Hypnotics	Benzodiazepines (BZD's)	Ativan®	loraze*pam*
			Dalmane®	furaze*pam*
			Halcion®	triazo*lam*
			Klonopin®	clonaze*pam*
			ProSom®	estazo*lam*
			Restoril®	temaze*pam*
			Serax®	oxaze*pam*
			Valium®	diaze*pam*
			Xanax®	alprazo*lam*
-pramine	Antidepressants	Tricyclic Antidepressants (TCA's)	Anafranil®	clomi*pramine*
			Norpramin®	desi*pramine*
			Tofranil®	imi*pramine*
-triptyline	Antidepressants	Tricyclic Antidepressants (TCA's)	Elavil®	ami*triptyline*
			Pamelor®	nor*triptyline*
			Vivactil®	pro*triptyline*
-ine	Antidepressants	Selective Serotonin Reuptake Inhibitors (SSRI's)	Paxil®	paroxet*ine*
			Prozac®	fluoxet*ine*
			Zoloft®	sertral*ine*

-one	Anti-inflammatory	Corticosteroids	Aristocort®, Kenalog®	triamcinolone
			Celestone®	betamethasone
			Cortef®, Hydrocortone®, Solu-Cortef®	hydrocortisone
			Cortone®	cortisone
			Decadron®	dexamethasone
			Delta-Cortef®, Prelone®, Pediapred®, Orapred®	prednisolone
			Deltasone®	prednisone
			Florinef®	fludrocortisone
			Solu-Medrol®, Medrol®, Depo-Medrol®	methylprednisolone
-steride	Benign Prostatic Hyperplasia (BPH)	5α-Reductase Inhibitors	Avodart®	dutasteride
			Proscar®	finasteride
-nacin	Overactive Bladder and Incontinence	Anticholinergics	Enablex®	darifenacin
			Vesicare®	Solifenacin
-fil	Erectile Dysfunction	PDE5-Inhibitors	Cialis®	tadalafil
			Levitra®	vardenafil
			Viagra®	sildenafil
-terol	Pulmonary	β-agonists	Foradil®	formoterol
			Maxair®	pirbuterol
			Proventil®, Ventolin®, Volmax®	albuterol
			Serevent®	salmeterol
			Xopenex®	levalbuterol
-mide, -nide	Antihypertensive	Diuretics	Lasix®	furosemide
			Bumex®	bumetamide
			Demadex®	torsemide
			Lozol®	indapamide

Exception:
- Clindamycin (Cleocin) is not a macrolide. It is a Lincomycin.

Practice Questions # 1

Match the drug class with a specific drug.

A. Macrolide
B. Tetracycline
C. Fluoroquinolone
D. Cephalosporin
E. Penicillin
F. Anti-Herpetic
G. ACE inhibitors
H. ARB
I. Alpha 1 receptor blocker
J. Beta-blocker
K. Calcium channel blocker
L. HMG-CoA reductase inhibitor
M. Thiazolidinedione
N. Meglitinide
O. Bisphosphonate
P. H2-Receptor antagonist
Q. 5-HT 1 receptor antagonist
R. Benzodiazepine

___ 1. Temazepam
___ 2. Ranitidine
___ 3. Starlix®
___ 4. Pravastatin
___ 5. Azithromycin
___ 6. Ciprofloxacin
___ 7. Amoxicillin
___ 8. Enalapril
___ 9. Doxazosin
___ 10. Felodipine
___ 11. Avandia®
___ 12. Minocycline
___ 13. Zolmitriptan
___ 14. Cefadroxil
___ 15. Alendronate
___ 16. Valacyclovir
___ 17. Irbesartan
___ 18. Bisoprolol

Answers Practice Questions #1
1.R 2.P 3.N 4.L 5.A 6.C 7.E 8.G 9.I 10.K 11.M 12.B 13.Q 14.D 15.O 16.F 17.H 18.J

Practice Questions # 2
Match the drug class with the suffix or prefix.

A.	Macrolide	___ 1.	-sartan
B.	Tetracycline	___ 2.	-cyclovir
C.	Fluoroquinolone	___ 3.	-dronate
D.	Cephalosporin	___ 4.	-statin
E.	Penicillin	___ 5.	-cillin
F.	Anti-Herpetic	___ 6.	-tidine
G.	ACE inhibitors	___ 7.	-dipine
H.	ARB	___ 8.	-glinide
I.	Alpha 1 receptor blocker	___ 9.	ceph-
J.	Beta-blocker	___ 10.	-triptan
K.	Calcium channel blocker	___ 11.	-olol
L.	HMG-CoA reductase inhibitor	___ 12.	-floxacin
M.	Thiazolidinedione	___ 13.	-lam
N.	Meglitinide	___ 14.	-osin
O.	Bisphosphonate	___ 15.	-cycline
P.	H2-Receptor antagonist	___ 16.	-glitazone
Q.	5-HT 1 receptor antagonist	___ 17.	-pril
R.	Benzodiazepine	___ 18.	-mycin

Answers Practice Questions # 2
1.H 2.F 3.O 4.L 5.E 6.P 7.K 8.N 9.D 10.Q 11.J 12.C 13.R 14.I 15.B 16.M 17.G 18.A

Practice Questions # 3
Match the drug category or disease state with a specific drug. (may use an answer multiple times)

A.	Hypertension	___ 1. Doxycycline	___ 16. Dutasteride		
B.	Anti-Inflammatory	___ 2. Albuterol	___ 17. Simvastatin		
C.	Antiviral	___ 3. Diazepam	___ 18. Nifedipine		
D.	Pulmonary Disease	___ 4. Ranitidine	___ 19. Amoxicillin		
E.	Benign Prostatic Hyperplasia	___ 5. Accupril	___ 20. Tamsulosin		
F.	Antiulcer	___ 6. Amitriptyline	___ 21. Ciprofloxacin		
G.	Antidepressant	___ 7. Fluoxetine	___ 22. Lansoprazole		
H.	Antibiotic	___ 8. Clonazepam	___ 23. Hydrocortisone		
I.	Hyperlipidemia	___ 9. Sumitriptan	___ 24. Alendronate		
J.	Diabetes	___ 10. Clarithromycin			
K.	Migraine	___ 11. Losartan			
L.	Antianxiety	___ 12. Sildenafil			
M.	Osteoporosis	___ 13. Darifenacin			
N.	Incontinence	___ 14. Cefuroxime			
O.	Erectile Dysfunction	___ 15. Atenolol			

Answers Practice Questions # 3
1.H 2.D 3.L 4.F 5.A 6.G 7.G 8.L 9.K 10.H 11.A 12.O 13.N 14.H 15.A 16.E 17.I 18.A 19.H 20.E 21.H 22.F 23.B 24.M

COMMON DRUGS

C
H
A
P
T
E
R
3

COMMON DRUGS

I. Endocrine and Metabolic

A. Diabetes Mellitus (DM)

Diabetes can be classified as type I, type II, and gestational. Gestational diabetes will not be covered in this book.

1. Type 1 diabetes (IDDM- Insulin dependent diabetes mellitus)

Type 1 diabetes is usually **diagnosed in early childhood**. The **body produces no insulin** due to the autoimmune degradation of beta cells in the pancreas and islet cells, which renders the patient insulin dependent. Being insulin dependent requires the **patient to receive insulin daily**. There are many different types of insulin, such as rapid acting, short acting, intermediate acting and long acting. Most oral medications work by either **stimulating** the production of insulin or by **prohibiting** the release of glucose into the body. Type I diabetics have no insulin being produced which causes an excess of glucose in the body; therefore giving oral medication to a type I diabetic is generally not proper treatment.

- Insulin vials are dispensed in units (u) per milliliter (ml) with a usual concentration of 100 units per ml. A 10 ml bottle would contain 1000 units of insulin (100 u x 10 = 1000 u).
- Most insulin is given subcutaneously (SC or SQ- directly under the skin). SC sites include **abdomen, upper arm**, and **thigh**. Do not give injections at the same site every time. It is important to **rotate sites**.
- Needles range in length from 3/8 to 5/8-inch (length of the needle used depends on the weight of the patient). Obese patients require a long needle due to excess subcutaneous tissue and young, thin patients with little subcutaneous tissue require shorter needles.
- The gauge of the needle represents the thickness of the needle. The gauge can range from 25 to 31. The higher the gauge, the thinner the needle. (i.e. 25 gauge is thicker than 31 gauge).
- Syringe sizes are 3/10 cc (30 units), 1/2 cc (50 units), and 1 cc (100 units). If a patient is injecting 20 units per dose a 30-unit syringe would be used. If a patient is injecting 45 units per dose then a 50-unit syringe should be used.
- Insulin can be administered by injection or oral inhalation. Injectable forms include shots, IV drips, pens and pumps. Exubera is an oral **inhalation** insulin powder.

Insulin Types

Rapid Acting

Generic	Brand
Insulin lispro	Humalog
Insulin aspart	Novolog
Insulin glulisine	Apidra
Insulin human	Exubera (inhalation)

Short Acting

Generic	Brand
Insulin regular	Humulin R, Novolin R

Intermediate Acting

Generic	Brand
Insulin isophane (NPH)	Humulin N, Novolin N
Insulin zinc suspension	Lente

Long Acting

Generic	Brand
Insulin glargine	Lantus
Insulin detemir	Levemir

Combinations

Generic	Brand
Insulin aspart protamine/ insulin aspart	Novolog Mix 70/30
Insulin lispro protamine/ insulin lispro	Humalog Mix 75/25
Insulin isophane (NPH) / insulin regular(R)	Humulin 70/30

Non-Insulin injectables

Generic	Brand
Exenatide	Byetta
Pramlintide	Symlin

Quick Facts

- Regular insulin, Lispro (Humalog) and Aspart (Novolog) insulins are **clear** and **colorless** solutions, which can be given SC or **IV** (notice all clear insulins are rapid acting, EXCEPT Lantus, which is long acting). All other insulins are suspensions and are therefore cloudy and can ONLY be given SC.
- Do not mix Glargine (Lantus) with any other insulin.
- Exubera is the **only oral inhalation insulin** on the market.
- Insulin at room temperature burns less than cold insulin, but room temperature insulin will expire in 28-30 days.
- Insulin is generally dispensed in 100 units/ml. A 10 ml vial contains 1000 units.
- Insulin is a string of amino acids. There are three types of insulin: **beef, pork or biosynthetic human insulin.**
- The only insulins that **Do Not** require a prescription are Humulin or Novolin N, R, 70/30, and lente insulins.

2. Type 2 diabetes (NIDDM- Non-Insulin dependent diabetes mellitus)

Type 2 diabetes is usually caused by **lifestyle choices** (obesity and/or sedentary lifestyle). Depending on the severity of the patient's diabetes, it can be treated by oral medications alone, or with a combination of oral medication and insulin.

Oral Medications

1. Sulfonylureas: suffix is *-ide*

These medications increase beta cell insulin secretion from the pancreas, decrease the amount of glucose released from the liver, and increase the sensitivity of insulin at peripheral target sites.

Generic	Brand
Tolbutam*ide*	Orinase
Acetohexam*ide*	Dymelor
Tolazam*ide*	Tolinase
Chlorpropam*ide*	Diabinese
Glybur*ide*	Diabeta, Micronase, Glynase
Glipiz*ide*	Glucotrol
Glimepir*ide*	Amaryl

2. Biguanides

Metformin works by increasing the peripheral muscle uptake of glucose and also inhibits the release of glucose from the liver.

Generic	Brand
Metformin	Glucophage

Quick Facts

- Metformin has a **black box warning** about the possibility of lactic acidosis.
- A common side effect of metformin is weight loss.
- Metformin is contraindicated in patients with congestive heart failure (CHF) and patients greater than 80 years of age.
- Metformin tablets have a fishy odor.

3. Alphaglucosidase inhibitors

These medications work by slowing down the breakdown of complex carbohydrates into glucose.

Generic	Brand
Acarbose	Precose
Miglitol	Glyset

Quick Facts

- Side effect is flatulence (gas).
- Do not take OTC Beano with alphaglucosidase inhibitors because they have opposite mechanisms of action.

4. Thiazolidinediones: suffix is –*glitazone*

These medications enhance the ability of insulin to work on the liver, muscle and fat tissue. It also inhibits the release of glucose from the liver.

Generic	Brand
Rosi*glitazone*	Avandia
Pio*glitazone*	Actos

5. Meglitinide: suffix is –*glinide*

These medications stimulate the release of insulin from the pancreas, but are glucose dependant.

Generic	Brand
Repa*glinide*	Prandin
Nate*glinide*	Starlix

Quick Facts

- Since the effectiveness of these medications is glucose dependant, it is necessary for the patient to take these medications 15 to 30 minutes before a meal.
- Meglitinides should not be taken in combination with Sulfonylureas because of similar mechanisms of action.

6. DPP-4 inhibitor

This medication works by increasing the release of insulin and decreasing the levels of glucagon in circulation through a glucose dependant manner.

Generic	Brand
Sitagliptin	Januvia

7. Combinations:

Generic	Brand
Glyburide/Metformin	Glucovance

Pioglitazone/Metformin	Actosplus met
Rosiglitazone/Metformin	Avandamet
Glipizine/Metformin	Metaglip

Quick Facts

- All of these oral medications can be used in combination with each other and with insulin. The **only exception** to this rule is that Metglitinides cannot be used with Sulfonylureas because of similar mechanisms of action.
- People with congestive heart failure should **not** take metformin.
- A blood glucose monitor gives the reading of a patient's blood glucose level at that moment. Testing blood **HbA1c** is a measure of glucose control over a **3 month** period. The HbA1c goal of a diabetic is to be below 7.
- **Hyperglycemia** is an excess of glucose in the blood and **hypoglycemia** is the lack of sufficient glucose in the blood.
- Glucagon injection, glucose tablets or glucose gel are used when a patient develops **low** blood sugar (hypoglycemia).

Diabetes Questions

1. How many days will it take a patient injecting 23 units of Humulin R insulin daily to complete a 10 ml vial?
   - a. 30 days
   - b. 23 days
   - c. 43 days
   - d. 14 days
2. Which size needle and syringe would a very thin patient use if injecting 23 units of insulin daily?
   - a. 1 cc short 25 gauge
   - b. 1/3 cc short 30 gauge
   - c. 1/2 cc long 30 gauge
   - d. 1/3 cc long 25 gauge
3. Glucagon is used _____.
   - a. When a patient has high blood sugar (hyperglycemia).
   - b. As a substitute for sugar in their diets.
   - c. When a patient has low blood sugar (hypoglycemia).
   - d. Daily with insulin injections to prevent hypoglycemia.
4. Type 1 diabetics would not use which medication?
   - a. Lantus
   - b. Glucagon
   - c. Glucotrol
   - d. Lispro
5. Which insulin is cloudy?
   - a. Humulin R
   - b. Humulin N
   - c. Lantus
   - d. All the above are cloudy
6. Which statement is true regarding insulin and refrigeration?
   - a. Insulin should never be refrigerated.
   - b. Insulin should never be left outside of the refrigerator.
   - c. Insulin is good for approximately 28 days outside of refrigeration.
   - d. Insulin burns more when injected at room temperature.

7. Which statement is true regarding Type 2 diabetics?
>   a. Usually diagnosed during pregnancy.
>   b. Only use insulin.
>   c. Can use both insulin and oral medications.
>   d. All of the above.

8. Type 1 diabetics can increase their pancreatic output of insulin by changing their diet and exercise.
>   a. true
>   b. false

9. Which insulin comes in an inhalation dosage form?
>   a. Exubera
>   b. Lantus
>   c. Humalog
>   d. Humulin 70/30 mix

10. Which insulin can be given IV?
>   a. Humulin R
>   b. Humulin N
>   c. Lantus
>   d. Humalog mix 75/25

11. Which drug is used to treat diabetes?
>   a. Metformin
>   b. Synthroid
>   c. Coreg
>   d. Ritalin

12. Which class of drugs is used to treat diabetes?
>   a. Sulfonylureas
>   b. Ace inhibitors
>   c. Aminoglycosides
>   d. Tetracyclines

13. Glyburide is used to treat which disease?
>   a. Hyperlipidemia
>   b. Bipolar disorder
>   c. Depression
>   d. Diabetes mellitus

14. Insulin is used to treat which condition?
>   a. Hyperglycemia
>   b. Hypoglycemia
>   c. Hyperlipidemia
>   d. Hypercalcemia

15. Where is insulin stored in the pharmacy?
>   a. Freezer
>   b. Rerfrigerator
>   c. On a shelf at room temperature
>   d. None of the above

16. What is the proper temperature for insulin storage?
>   a. 10-20 degrees Fahrenheit
>   b. 53-63 degrees Fahrenheit
>   c. 45-55 degrees Fahrenheit
>   d. 36-46 degrees Fahrenheit

17. Hypoglycemia is defined as _____.
>   a. Elevated cholesterol
>   b. Low blood sugar
>   c. High blood sugar
>   d. Low calcium

18. Which type of diabetes is usually diagnosed in childhood?
    a. Type 2
    b. Type 1
    c. Gestational diabetes
    d. Type 4
19. Which type of diabetes is known as insulin dependent diabetes mellitus?
    a. Type 4
    b. Type 1
    c. Type A
    d. Type 2
20. How many units are in a standard bottle of Regular U-100 insulin?
    a. 10
    b. 50
    c. 100
    d. 1000
21. Humulin N is injected by which route of administration?
    a. IV
    b. IM
    c. SC
    d. IV Push
22. Which type of injection offers the quickest onset of action?
    a. IM
    b. SC
    c. IV
    d. ID
23. An HbA1C test will show glucose control over what period of time?
    a. 3 months
    b. 10 days
    c. 1 month
    d. 1 week
24. How long can insulin be left at room temperature before it must be discarded?
    a. Approximately 1 month
    b. Approximately 2 months
    c. Approximately 3 months
    d. Until the insulin reaches the expiration date listed on the bottle
25. Which of the following insulins has the longest duration of action?
    a. Lantus
    b. Humulin R
    c. Humalog
    d. Humulin N
26. Insulin injections should be given at the same injection site to maintain a constant level of absorption.
    a. True
    b. False

Diabetes Answers
1.c 2.b 3.c 4.c 5.b 6.c 7.c 8.b 9.a 10.a 11.a 12.a 13.d 14.a 15.b 16.d 17.b 18.b 19.b 20.d 21.c 22.c 23.a 24.a 25.a 26.b

B. Thyroid Drugs

These medications treat **hypothyroidism** (deficiency of thyroid hormone) and **hyperthyroidism** (excess of thyroid hormone).

Generic	Brand	Indication	Hormone	Notes
Levothyroxine	Levothroid, Levoxyl, Synthroid, Unithroid	Hypothyroidism	T4	
Thyroid desiccated	Armour Thyroid	Hypothyroidism	T4, T3	Natural from animal thyroid
Liothyronine	Cytomel	Hypothroidism	T3	
Liotrix	Thyrolar	Hypothroidism	T4, T3	Synthetic T4:T3 ratio of 4:1
Propylthiouracil	PTU(abbreviation)	HYPERthyroidism		
Methimazole	Tapazole	HYPERthyroidism		

Quick Facts

- Most thyroid medications are dispensed in mcg and mg except Armour Thyroid, which is dispensed in mg and grains.
- Propylthiouracil is used in pregnant women with **hyper**thyroidism.
- Do not take with antacids.

Thyroid Questions

1. Which drug treats hypothyroidism?
   - a. Propylthiouracil
   - b. Fluoxetine
   - c. Levothyroxine
   - d. Levodopa
2. What is the generic name for Synthroid?
   - a. Labetalol
   - b. Paroxetine
   - c. Levothyroxine
   - d. Carbamazepine
3. What is the abbreviation for propylthiouracil?
   - a. PCP
   - b. PCN
   - c. AZT
   - d. PTU
4. Which strength of Synthroid is correct?
   - a. 0.200 mg
   - b. 0.200 mcg
   - c. 0.200 g
   - d. 2 mcg
5. Armour Thyroid 1 grain is equivalent to how many milligrams?
   - a. 100 mcg
   - b. 100 mg
   - c. 60 mcg
   - d. 60 mg

Thyroid Answers

1. c 2. c 3. d 4. a 5. d

C. Osteoporosis Drugs

These medications treat and prevent osteoporosis. Osteoporosis is a condition that involves bone loss and the softening of bones, which can lead to bone fractures.

1. Bisphosphonates: suffix is *-dronate*

Generic	Brand	Route
Alen*dronate*	Fosamax	PO
Pami*dronate*	Aredia	PO
Eti*dronate*	Didronel	PO
Rise*dronate*	Actonel	PO
Tilu*dronate*	Skelid	PO
Iban*dronate*	Boniva	PO

Quick Facts

- Boniva is taken only **once a month.**
- Actonel 35 mg and Fosamax 35 mg and 70 mg are taken **once weekly.**
- Biphosphonates *"-dronates"* should be taken:
    - With 6-8 ounces of water.
    - First thing in the morning before eating or drinking anything (other than water).
    - Do not lie down, eat, drink (other than water), or take any other medication for at least 30 minutes after taking Bisphosphonates; this will reduce the risk of irritation and/or erosion of the esophagus.

2. Miscellaneous drugs

Generic	Brand	Route
Calcitonin-salmon	Miacalcin, Fortical	Intranasal

Quick Facts

- Miacalcin is stored in the pharmacy **refrigerator** prior to dispensing.
- It is an intranasal spray.
- The normal dosage is one spray in alternating nostrils everyday.

Osteoporosis Questions

1. How is Miacalcin stored prior to dispensing?
    - a. Refrigeration
    - b. Room temperature
    - c. Freezer
    - d. Separated from all other drugs
2. How is Miacalcin administered?
    - a. By mouth
    - b. Subcutaneously
    - c. Intranasal
    - d. Transdermal
3. What is the dosing frequency of Boniva?
    - a. Once monthly
    - b. Once daily
    - c. Every morning
    - d. Once weekly
4. How is Fosamax taken?
    - a. With food
    - b. With antacids
    - c. 30 minutes before breakfast and with water only
    - d. 30 minutes before bedtime

5. What is the dosing frequency of Fosamax 70mg?
   a. Once daily
   b. Once monthly
   c. Once weekly
   d. Twice weekly
6. Which drug is not used for osteoporosis?
   a. Alendronate
   b. Actonel
   c. Cyanocobalamin
   d. Miacalcin
7. Why should a patient not lie down after taking Biphosphonates?
   a. Diarrhea
   b. Erosion of the esophagus
   c. Decreased absorption of the medication
   d. None of the above

Osteoporosis Answers
1.a 2.c 3.a 4.c 5.c 6.c 7.b

II. Cardiovascular System

Hypertension (HTN)

Hypertension (high blood pressure) is caused by the resistance of blood flow through blood vessels. This resistance is determined by measuring systolic pressure (cardiac output) and diastolic pressure (peripheral resistance). The top number (120) is the systolic pressure and the bottom number (80) is the diastolic pressure. An ideal blood pressure reading is 120/80 mm Hg. HTN can be hereditary or due to lifestyle choices. There are many drugs, with different mechanisms of action that are used to control HTN.

- It is difficult to learn all of the brand and generic names for HTN medications. Pay close attention to the endings (suffixes) of the generic names. By knowing the suffixes, it is much easier to determine which class a drug belongs. **Be careful,** this applies **only** to generic suffixes, not to the brand suffixes.
- **Pseudoephedrine is contraindicated in patients with severe or uncontrolled hypertension.**

A. Anti-Hypertensive Drugs

1. Betablockers: suffix is *–olol* or *-lol*

Betablockers work in hypertensive patients by binding to Beta 1 receptors, which decreases heart rate, cardiac output, and causes relaxation of blood vessels.

Generic	Brand	Blocking Agent	Indications	Route
Acebut*olol*	Sectral	Beta 1	HTN, Arrhythmias	PO
Aten*olol*	Tenormin	Beta 1	HTN, Angina, Acute MI	PO IV
Betax*olol*	Kerlone	Beta 1	HTN	PO
Esm*olol*	Brevibloc	Beta 1	Supraventricular tachycardia, Sinus tachycardia	IV infusion
Metopr*olol* Metopr*olol*	Lopressor Toprol XL	Beta 1	HTN, Angina Pectoris, Acute MI	PO IV
Carte*olol*	Cartrol	Beta 1 Beta 2	HTN	PO
Nad*olol*	Corgard	Beta 1 Beta 2	HTN Angina Pectoris	PO

34

Penbut*olol*	Levatol	Beta 1 Beta 2	HTN	PO
Pind*olol*	Visken	Beta 1 Beta 2	HTN	PO
Propran*olol*	Inderal	Beta 1 Beta 2	HTN, Angina pectoris, Arrhythmias	PO
Sota*lol*	Betapace	Beta 1 Beta 2	Ventricular arrhythmias, Atrial fibrillation	PO
Tim*olol*	Blocadren	Beta 1 Beta 2	HTN	PO
Carvedi*lol*	Coreg	Beta 1 Beta 2 Alpha 1	HTN, CHF	PO
Labeta*lol*	Trandate, Normodyne	Beta 1 Beta 2 Alpha 1	HTN	PO IV

Quick Facts

- Be careful, it is easy to be tricked by names that look like they may be betablockers due to their -ol ending (e.g. the generic name for Ultram, is tramad**ol**, an analgesic; Tegret**ol**, an anticonvulsant, is the brand name for carbamazepine).
- Do not abruptly discontinue beta blockers.
- **Orthostatic hypotension** (lightheadedness upon standing) is a common side effect of betablockers.
- Beta 1 receptors are located in the heart and kidneys.
- Beta 2 receptors are located in the lungs, liver, pancreas and arteriolar smooth muscle.
- Since Beta 2 receptors are in the lungs and pancreas, they should be used very cautiously in patients with asthma, COPD (chronic obstructive pulmonary disease), and diabetes.
- Betablockers may be used alone or in combination with other hypertensive medications.

2. ACE inhibitors (ACEI's): suffix is *-pril*

These medications work by exerting their effects on the Renin Angiotensin System in the kidneys. Inhibiting angiotensin-converting enzyme (ACE) prevents the conversion of angiotensin I to angiotensin II. Angiotensin II is a potent vasoconstrictor. The reduction of angiotensin II also decreases aldosterone secretion and thus reduces sodium and water rentention. These actions lead to a reduction in blood pressure.

Generic	Brand	Indications	Route
Benaza*pril*	Lotensin	HTN	PO
Capto*pril*	Capoten	HTN, CHF	PO
Enala*pril*	Vasotec	HTN, CHF	PO
Enala*pril*	Enalaprilat	HTN	IV
Fosino*pril*	Monopril	HTN, CHF	PO
Linsino*pril*	Zestril, Prinivil	HTN, CHF	PO
Moexi*pril*	Univasc	HTN	PO
Perindo*pril*	Coversyl	HTN	PO
Quini*pril*	Accupril	HTN, CHF	PO
Rami*pril*	Altace	HTN, CHF	PO

- Common side effects of ACE inhibitors are **angioedema** and **dry cough.** The build-up of bradykinin causes the dry cough.
- Generally, ACE inhibitors are not used in pregnancy (category C in 1st trimester, category D in 2nd and 3rd trimesters).

3. Angiotensin II receptor antagonists (ARB's): suffix is *-sartan*

These medications work by exerting their effects on angiotensin II receptors. They block the vasoconstriction and the aldosterone secreting effects of angiotensin II; therefore, resulting in a reduction of blood pressure.

Generic	Brand	Indication	Route
Cande*sartan*	Atacand	HTN	PO
Epro*sartan*	Teveten	HTN	PO
Irbe*sartan*	Avapro	HTN	PO
Lo*sartan*	Cozaar	HTN	PO
Telmi*sartan*	Micardis	HTN	PO
Val*sartan*	Diovan	HTN	PO

Quick Facts
- Generally, Angiotensin II receptor antagonists are not used in pregnancy (category C in 1st trimester, category D in 2nd and 3rd trimesters).
- Although ACE inhibitors and Angiotensin II receptor antagonist's mechanisms of action are closely related, the advantages of the "sartans" (ARB's) are that there is no cough and less angioedema.

4. Calcium Channel Blockers (CCB's): suffix is generally *–dipine*

The antihypertensive action of CCB's is due due to the reduced influx of calcium into cardiac smooth muscle. This reduction of calcium influx causes blood vessel dilation (vasodilation) to the heart, therefore reducing blood pressure.

Generic	Brand	Indication	Route
Amlo*dipine*	Norvasc	HTN, Angina	PO
Bepridil	Bapadin	Angina	PO
Diltiazem	Cardizem, Cartia, Dilacor, Tiamate, Tiazac	HTN, Angina, Atrial fibrillation or flutter, Paroxysmal supraventricular tachycardia (PSVT)	PO IV
Felo*dipine*	Plendil	HTN, CHF	PO
Isra*dipine*	DynaCirc	HTN, CHF, Migraine Prophylaxis	PO
Nicar*dipine*	Cardene SR Cardene	HTN, Angina, Migraine Prohylaxis, CHF	PO IV
Nife*dipine*	Adalat, Procardia	HTN, Angina, Pulmonary hypertension, Migraine headaches, Raynaud's disease	PO
Nisol*dipine*	Sular	HTN	PO
Verapamil	Calan, Covera-HS, Isoptin, Verelan	Angina pectoris, HTN, PSVT, Atrial fibrillation or flutter.	PO IV

Quick Facts
- Constipation is a common side effect of Verapamil.
- Flushing, reflex tachycardia and edema are common side effects of Nifedipine.

5. Diuretics

The antihypertensive action of diuretics is through increased urinary excretion of sodium, chloride, potassium, and water.

a. Thiazides and Sulfonamides: suffix is generally *-thiazide*

Generic	Brand	Indication	Route
Hydrochlro*thiazide*	Hydrodiuril	HTN, Edema in CHF	PO, Solution
Chloro*thiazide*	Diuril	HTN, Edema in CHF	PO, IV
Methyclo*thiazide*	Enduron	HTN, Edema in CHF	PO
Hydroflume*thiazide*	Saluron, Diucardin	HTN, Edema in CHF	PO
Poly*thiazide*	Renese	HTN, Edema in CHF	PO
Indapamide	Lozol	HTN, Edema in CHF	PO
Metolazone	Zaroxolyn	HTN, Edema in CHF	PO
Quinethazone	Hydromox	HTN, Edema in CHF	PO

b. Loop diuretics: suffix is *–mide* or *-nide*

Generic	Brand	Indication	Route
Furose*mide*	Lasix	HTN, Edema	PO, Injection
Bumeta*nide*	Bumex	HTN, Edema	PO, Injection
Torse*mide*	Demadex	HTN, Edema	PO

Quick Facts

- Counsel patients to take diuretics in the morning due to increased urination.
- Potassium tablets (K-dur, Klor-Con, etc.) are usually taken with diuretics due to increased potassium excretion (potassium loss).

6. Alpha2-Adrenergic Agonists: suffix is *–dine* or *-cine*

Generic	Brand	Indication	Route
Cloni*dine*	Catapres	HTN	PO, Transdermal, Epidural Transfusion
Dexmedetomi*dine*	Precedex	Sedation	IV
Guanabenz	Wytensin	HTN	PO
Tizani*dine*	Zanaflex	Muscle relaxant	PO
Guanfa*cine*	Tenex	HTN	PO

7. Alpha-Adrenergic Inhibitors

Generic	Brand	Indication	Route
Methyldopa	Aldomet	HTN	PO, IV

Quick Facts

- Methyldopa is commonly used to treat hypertension in pregnant women.

8. Alpha1 Adrenergic Blockers: suffix is *-osin*

Generic	Brand	Indication	Route
Doxaz*osin*	Cardura	HTN, BPH	PO
Teraz*osin*	Hytrin	HTN, BPH	PO
Praz*osin*	Minipress	BPH	PO
Alfuz*osin*	Uroxatral	BPH	PO
Tamsul*osin*	Flomax	BPH	PO

B. Antiarrhythmic Drugs

These medications treat irregular heart beats such as tachycardia, fibrillation, and flutter.

Class I

Generic	Brand
Moricizine	Ethmozine

Class Ia

Generic	Brand
Disopyramide	Norpace
Quinidine	Quinidex, Quinaglute
Procainamide	Ponestyl

Class Ib

Generic	Brand
Phenytoin	Dilantin, Phenytek
Mexiletine	Mexitil
Lidocaine	Xylocaine

Class Ic

Generic	Brand
Flecainide	Tambocor
Propafenone	Rythmol

Class II- betablockers

Generic	Brand
Esmo**lol**	Brevibloc
Acebut**olol**	Sectral
Sota**lol**	Betapace
Propran**olol**	Inderal

Class III

Generic	Brand
Amiodarone	Cordarone, Pacerone
Dofetilide	Tikosyn
Bretylium	Bretylol
Sotalol	Betapace
Ibutilide	Corvert

Class IV

Generic	Brand
Digoxin	Lanoxin
Adenosine	Adenocard
Verapamil	Calan, Isoptin

C. Vasodilators

Generic	Brand	Route
Nitroglycerin	Nitrostat, Nitroquick, Minitran, Nitro-Bid, Nitro-Dur, Nitro-Tab, Nitrek,	PO, IV, Sublingual, Translingual spray, Topical ointment, Transdermal
Isosorbide Dinitrate	Isordi, Dilatrate-SR, Isochron	PO, Sublingual, Chewable
Isosorbide Mononitrate	Imdur, Ismo, Monoket	PO
Amyl Nitrite	Isoamyl Nitrate	Nasal inhalation
Nitroprusside	Nitropress	IV
Hydralazine	Apo-Hydralazine, Apresoline	PO, IM, IV
Dipyridamole	Persantine	PO, IV
Minoxidil	Loniten, Rogaine	Solution (Rogaine), Tablet (Loniten)
Treprostinil	Remodulin	SC, IV

Quick Facts
- Nitroglycerin is **contraindicated** with Viagra, Cialis, or Levitra due to possible prolonged **hypo**tension.
- Nitroglycerin patches should be removed for 12 hours each day to provide a nitrate-free period.
- Nitroglycerin sublingual tablets **do not** require child proof packaging.

D. Anticoagulants: suffix is *-arin* or *-in*

These medications treat or prevent venous thrombosis, stroke or myocardial infarction by slowing down the blood clotting process. Patients taking anticoagulants (also called blood-thinners) must be monitored closely due to the risk of increased bleeding.

Generic	Brand	Route
Hep*arin*	HepFlush-10, Hep-lock	IV
Antithromb*in* III	Thrombate III	Injection, Powder for reconstitution
Warf*arin*	Coumadin, Jantoven	PO, Injection, Powder for reconstitution
Bivalirub*in*	Angiomax	IV
Lepirud*in*	Refludan	Injection, Powder for reconstitution
Daltep*arin*	Fragmin	Injection
Enoxap*arin*	Lovenox	Injection
Tinzap*arin*	Innohep	Injection
Fondap*arin*ux	Arixtra	Injection

Quick Facts
- Warfarin is **contraindicated** with other drugs that prevent blood clotting, such as aspirin and NSAIDs (Ibuprofen, Naproxen and Ketoprofen etc.), unless the patient is being advised and monitored by their physician.
- If a patient is on warfarin and needs an antipyretic (fever-reducer), they should be counseled to take acetaminophen (Tylenol), which is an analgesic/antipyretic (pain reducer and fever reducer), and has no blood thinning properties.
- Warfarin is a pregnancy **category X.**
- A major side effect of Warfarin is bruising and increased bleeding time.
- Warfarin dosage is calculated based on the INR test.
- Maintenance daily dosing of Warfarin ranges from 2 mg to 10 mg.
- Vitamin K (Phytonadione) is used as a clotting factor if a patient has overdosed on Warfarin.

E. Cholesterol and Lipid Lowering Drugs
These medications treat elevated cholesterol and triglyceride levels.
1. HMG-CoA reductase inhibitors: suffix is *-statins*

Generic	Brand	Route
Lova*statin*	Mevacor	PO
Simva*statin*	Zocor	PO
Prava*statin*	Pravachol	PO
Fluva*statin*	Lescol	PO
Atorva*statin*	Lipitor	PO
Rosuva*statin*	Crestor	PO

Quick Facts
- Pregnancy **category X.**
- Common side effects of HMG-CoA reductase inhibitors include leg cramps, muscle degeneration (rhabdomyolysis) and liver damage.
- Liver function tests (LFTs) must be done to monitor for possible liver damage.
- "Statins" are usually taken in the evening.

2. Triglyceride Reducers

Generic	Brand	Route
Gemfibrozil	Lopid	PO
Fenofibrate	Tricor	PO

Quick Facts
- Side effects are usually GI related and leg cramps.

3. Miscellaneous Cholesterol Lowering Drugs

Generic	Brand	Route
Cholestyramine	Questran, Prevalite	PO (powder)
Niacin	Vitamin B3	PO
Colestipol	Colestid	PO
Omacor	Omega3 fatty acids	PO
Ezetimibe	Zetia	PO

Quick Facts
- The side effect of Niacin is **flushing** which can be prevented by pre-treating with aspirin 1/2 to 1 hour before taking Niacin.

Cardiovascular Questions
1. Which of the following drugs is a betablocker?
   - a. Tramadol
   - b. Enalapril
   - c. Atenolol
   - d. Amlodipine

2. Which suffix is generally associated with betablockers?
     a. –pam
     b. –azole
     c. –olol
     d. –pril

3. Which suffix is generally associated with ACE inhibitors?
     a. –olol
     b. –cycline
     c. –mycin
     d. –pril

4. Which condition is a diuretic used to treat?
     a. Edema
     b. Hyperlipidemia
     c. Pyschosis
     d. Depression

5. Which drug is exempt from childproof closures?
     a. Oral contraceptives
     b. Sublingual nitroglycerin tablets
     c. Amoxicillin suspension
     d. Temazepam

6. Nitroglycerin sublingual must be stored in its original glass bottle.
     a. True
     b. False

7. What color is used to protect prescription vials from sunlight?
     a. Red
     b. Green
     c. Black
     d. Amber

8. Viagra is contraindicated with which of the following drugs?
     a. Benzodiazepines
     b. Loop diuretics
     c. Nitroglycerin
     d. Antidepressants

9. Coumadin is contraindicated with which of the following drugs?
     a. Percodan
     b. Percocet
     c. Amitriptyline
     d. Potassium chloride

10. Coumadin is in which pregnancy category?
     a. C
     b. A
     c. D
     d. X

11. Which of the following drugs is not an anticoagulant?
     a. Heparin
     b. Warfarin
     c. Levothyroxine
     d. Lovenox

12. Lovenox is taken by mouth.
     a. True
     b. False

13. Which of the following drugs should not be given to patients with hypertension?
    a. Furosemide
    b. Pseudoephedrine
    c. Amoxicillin
    d. Acetaminophen
14. Which of the following dosage forms is available for nitroglycerin?
    a. Sublingual tablet
    b. Capsule
    c. Transdermal patch
    d. Ointment
    e. All of the above
15. Which of the following vitamins is also known as Niacin?
    a. Vitamin B6
    b. Vitamin C
    c. Vitamin E
    d. Vitamin B3
16. Lovastatin is in which pregnancy category?
    a. X
    b. A
    c. B
    d. D
17. Diuretics should be taken in the morning.
    a. True
    b. False
18. Which one of the following statements is not a counseling point for a patient taking Lipitor?
    a. May cause leg cramps
    b. May cause dry cough
    c. Do not take if pregnant or planning to become pregnant
    d. Take with plenty of water
19. Which of the following drugs is an HMG Co-A reductase inhibitor?
    a. Captopril
    b. Atenolol
    c. Gemfibrozil
    d. Lovastatin
20. Which of the following drugs has a major side effect of dry cough?
    a. Valsartan
    b. Lisinopril
    c. Nadolol
    d. Flecainide
21. Which of the following drugs is not used to treat hypertension?
    a. Zetia
    b. Propranolol
    c. Verapamil
    d. Hydrochlorothiazide
22. What is the generic name for Norvasc?
    a. Amiodarone
    b. Propafenone
    c. Amlodipine
    d. Clonidine

23. Which of the following drugs is not a diuretic?
>   a. Torsemide
>   b. Hydrochlorothiazide
>   c. Niacin
>   d. Indapamide

24. Which drug class does Verapamil belong?
>   a. Calcium channel blocker
>   b. Betablocker
>   c. ACE inhibitor
>   d. Diuretic

25. Which statement is true regarding Coumadin?
>   a. Coumadin is considered a blood thinner
>   b. Coumadin is pregnancy category X
>   c. Coumadin dosing is based on INR testing
>   d. All of the above

Cardiovascular Answers

1.c 2.c 3.d 4.a 5.b 6.a 7.d 8.c 9.a 10.d 11.c 12.b 13.b 14.e 15.d 16.a 17.a 18.b 19.d 20.b 21.a 22.c 23.c 24.a 25.d

III. Central Nervous System Drugs

A. Antidepressants

1. Tricyclic Antidepressants (TCA's): suffix is *–triptyline* or *-pramine*

These drugs inhibit the reuptake of serotonin and norepineprine.

Generic	Brand	Route
Ami*triptyline*	Elavil	PO, Injectable
Desi*pramine*	Norpramin	PO
Amoxapine	Anafranil	PO
Imi*pramine*	Tofranil	PO
Doxepin	Sinequan	PO, Liquid
Nor*triptyline*	Pamelor	PO, Liquid
Trimi*pramine*	Surmontil	PO
Pro*triptyline*	Vivactil	PO

Quick Facts

- A common side effect of TCA's is sedation, and therefore they may be used to treat insomnia.

2. Selective Serotonin Reuptake Inhibitors (SSRI's): suffix is *–pram* or *-ine*

These medications work by inhibiting the reuptake of serotonin into the brain, therefore increasing the levels of serotonin which can cause mood elevation.

Generic	Brand	Route
Citalo*pram*	Celexa	PO, Liquid
Escitalo*pram*	Lexapro	PO
Fluoxet*ine*	Prozac	PO, Liquid
Fluvoxam*ine*	Luvox	PO
Paroxet*ine*	Paxil	PO, Liquid
Sertral*ine*	Zoloft	PO, Liquid

Quick Facts

- Side effects of SSRI's include suicidal tendencies and sexual dysfunction.
- It may take up to 6 weeks before the full therapeutic effects of these medications are achieved.

43

3. Serotonin and Norepinephrine Reuptake inhibitors (SNRIs)

Generic	Brand	Route
Duloxetine	Cymbalta	PO
Venlafaxine	Effexor	PO

4. Weak Dopamine, Serotonin and Norepinephrine Reuptake Inhibitors

Generic	Brand	Route
Bupropion	Wellbutrin, Zyban	PO

Quick Facts
- This medication may be used as an antidepressant and also for smoking cessation.

5. Serotonin Receptor Antagonists: suffix is *-odone*

Generic	Brand	Route
Traz*odone*	Desyrel	PO
Nefaz*odone*	Serzone	PO

6. Monoamine Oxidase Inhibitors (MAOI's)

Generic	Brand	Route
Phenelzine	Nardil	PO
Tranylcypromine	Pamate	PO
Isocarboxazid	Marplan	PO

Quick Facts
- MAOI's interact with foods containing tyramine and with foods that are processed using bacteria and microbes. The interaction can cause a severe hypertensive crisis known as the "Wine and Cheese Effect."
- Tyramine containing products include caffeine (coffee, tea and chocolate), yeast (beer and wine) and bacteria and/or fungi (cheeses, soy sauce, yogurt and avocados).
- MAOI's are rarely used in the treatment of depression due to the many food and drug interactions. They are considered last resort medications.

B. Migraine Drugs: suffix is *-triptan*
These medications treat acute migraine attacks.

Gereric	Brand	Route
Almo*triptan*	Axert	PO
Ele*triptan*	Relpax	PO
Frova*triptan*	Frova	PO
Nara*triptan*	Amerge	PO
Riza*triptan*	Maxalt	PO
Zolmi*triptan*	Zomig	PO, Nasal
Sumi*triptan*	Imitrex	PO, SC, Nasal

Quick Facts
- Must wait two hours before taking a second dose.
- **Do not** use in patients with coronary artery disease

C. Antipsychotics

These medications treat schizophrenia and mania. They work by decreasing the amount of dopamine in the central nervous system.

Generic	Brand	Route
Aripiprazole	Abilify	PO
Clozapine	Clozaril	PO
Chlorpromazine	Thorazine	PO, Injection, Suppositories
Haloperidol	Haldol	PO, Injectable
Fluphenazine	Pemitil, Prolixin	PO, Injectable
Loxapine	Loxitane	PO, Injectable
Mesoridazine	Serentil	PO, Injectable
Olanzapine	Zyprexa	PO, Injection
Molindone	Moban	PO
Perphenazine	Trilafon	PO, Injection
Pimozide	Orap	PO
Quetiapine	Seroquel	PO
Risperidone	Risperdal	PO, Injection
Thioridazine	Mellaril	PO
Thiothixene	Navane	PO, Powder for injection
Trifluoperazine	Stelazine	PO, Injection
Ziprasidone	Geodon	PO, Injection

Quick Facts

- A pharmacy must be registered to dispense Clozapine. White blood cell counts must be monitored due to the possibility of developing agranulocytosis.
- It may take up to 6 weeks before the therapeutic effects of these medications are achieved.
- Several of these drugs are also used to treat nausea and vomiting.
- There are two **serious** side effects that may occur when taking these medications long term. If these side effects are noticed, the medication **must** be stopped immediately.
    - **Tardive dyskinesia:** Involves involuntary movement of tongue, head, jaw and other various facial muscles. These effects may or may not be reversible. The reversibility is dependant upon how long the patient has been taking the medication and the severity of the tardive dyskinesia.
    - **Extrapyramidal effects:** These symptoms are Parkinson-like in nature and include shaking, shuffling when walking and drooling. These effects usually stop once the medication is discontinued or the dosage is lowered.

D. Seizure Drugs

These medications treat seizures (epilepsy) or convulsions.

Generic	Brand	Route
Phenytoin	Dilantin, Phenytek	PO, Injection
Carbamazepine	Tegretol	PO
Oxcarbazepine	Trileptal	PO
Gabapentin	Neurontin	PO
Pregabalin CV	Lyrica	PO
Lamotrigine	Lamictal	PO

Levetiracetam	Keppra	PO
Primidone	Mysoline	PO
Topiramate	Topamax	PO
Valproic Acid	Depakote	PO
Phenobarbital CIV	Luminal sodium	PO, Injection

E. Anxiety & Hypnotic Drugs

1. Antianxiety (Benzodiazepines): suffixes are generally *–pam* or *–lam*

These medications treat anxiety, panic disorder, insomnia, and muscle spasms.

Generic	Brand	Route
Alprazo*lam* CIV	Xanax	PO
Clorazepate CIV	Tranxene	PO
Chlordiazepoxide CIV	Librium	PO
Clonaze*pam* CIV	Klonopin	PO
Diaze*pam* CIV	Valium	PO, Injection
Loraze*pam* CIV	Ativan	PO, Injection
Oxaze*pam* CIV	Serax	PO

Quick Facts

- Buspirone (Buspar) – It is a non-benzodiazepine drug used to treat anxiety. It is not a controlled drug substance.
- All **benzodiazepines** are controlled drug substances **CIV**.
- All drugs in this class usually cause sedation and impair motor function. Therefore, the patient should not drink or drive while taking these medications.
- Clorazepate and Chlordiazepoxide are the only two benzodiazepines that do not end in –pam or –lam.

2. Hypnotic (sleep inducing) (Benzodiazepines)

Generic	Brand	Route
Estazo*lam* CIV	Prosom	PO
Fluraze*pam* CIV	Dalmane	PO
Temaze*pam* CIV	Restoril	PO
Triazo*lam* CIV	Halcion	PO

Quick Facts

- Midazolam (Versed) – CIV – It is an injectable benzodiazepine used for pre-operative sedation and anesthesia during short procedures (a.k.a. conscious sedation).

3. Miscellaneous Hypnotic (Non-benzodiazepines)

Generic	Brand	Route
Zolpidem CIV	Ambien	PO
Zaleplon CIV	Sonata	PO
Ramelteon	Rozerem	PO
Chloral Hydrate CIV	Somnote	PO

| Escopiclone CIV | Lunesta | PO |

Quick Facts
- Ramelteon (Rozerem) is the only prescription hypnotic drug that is not a controlled drug substance.

F. Pain Relievers (Analgesics)

1. Narcotic Analgesics

These medications treat mild, moderate, severe acute and chronic pain.

Generic	Brand	Route
APAP/Codeine CIII	Tylenol#3, Tylenol#4	PO
Fentanyl CII	Sublimaze, Duragesic, Actiq	Injection, transdermal, lozenge
Hydromorphone CII	Dilaudid	PO, Injection
Meperidine CII	Demerol	PO, Injection
Methadone CII	Dolophine	PO
Morphine CII	MSIR, MS Contin	PO, Injection
Oxycodone CII	Oxycontin, OxyIR	PO
APAP/Oxycodone CII	Percocet, Tylox	PO
ASA/Oxycodone CII	Percodan	PO
APAP/ Hydrocodone CIII	Lortab, Vicodin, Norco, Lorcet	PO
APAP/ Propoxyphene CIV	Darvocet N-100	PO
Butorphanol CIV	Stadol	IV, Nasal
Pentazocine/Naloxone CIV	Talwin NX	PO

Quick Facts
- Adverse effects include nausea, vomiting, sedation, constipation, and respiratory depression.
- Counseling points should include: 1) Take these medications with food to decrease nausea and vomiting. 2) Take with a stool softener. 3) Do not drive or drink alcohol while taking these medications.

2. NSAID's (Nonsteroidal Anti-Inflammatory Drugs)

These medications treat pain and inflammation associated with rheumatoid and osteoarthritis. They are also used for headaches, menstrual cramps, and general inflammation.

Generic	Brand	Route
Diclofenac	Cataflam, Voltaren	PO
Etodolac	Lodine	PO
Fenoprofen	Nalfon	PO
Flurbiprofen	Ansaid	PO
Ibuprofen	Advil, Motrin	PO
Indomethacin	Indocin	PO, **Suppository, Injection**
Ketoprofen	Oruvail, Orudis	PO
Ketorolac	Toradol	PO, **Injection**
Celecoxib	Celebrex	PO

Mefenamic Acid	Ponstel	PO
Meloxicam	Mobic	PO
Nabumetone	Relafen	PO
Naproxen	Anaprox DS, Naprosyn, Aleve	PO
Oxaprozin	Daypro	PO
Piroxicam	Feldene	PO
Sulindac	Clinoril	PO
Tolmetin	Tolectin DS	PO

Quick Facts

- Ketorolac (Toradol) is indicated for the management of moderately severe pain. It has a **black box warning to NOT** exceed using this medication greater than 5 days due to the possibility of GI bleeding, perforation or peptic ulcer. The 5 day maximum includes both parenteral and oral combined treatments.
- Celecoxib (Celebrex) is a COX-2 inhibitor; this drug causes less GI side effects than NSAID's. It is usually chosen over NSAID's in patients that have a history of GI problems. Other COX-2 inhibitors (Vioxx, Bextra) were recalled and permanently taken off the market due to patients developing cardiac problems.
- The adverse effects of NSAID's usually relate to the GI tract (dyspepsia, heartburn and nausea). These effects can be minimized by taking NSAID's with food and/or antacids.
- Many of the NSAID's are enteric coated to reduce GI side effects.
- Indomethacin (Indocin) is the only NSAID that comes in a suppository dosage form. Indomethacin is usually used in the treatment of gout.
- Indomethacin and Ketorlac are the **only injectable** NSAID's.

G. Antiparkinson Drugs

These medications treat Parkinson's disease. Parkinson's disease is a neurological disease caused by an imbalance of the neurotransmitters acetylcholine and dopamine. In Parkinson's disease there is an excess of acetylcholine and a deficiency of dopamine, which causes rigidity and tremors.

Generic	Brand	Action
Benztropine	Cogentin	Anti-cholinergic
Diphenhydramine	Benadryl	Anti-cholinergic
Trihexyphenidyl		Anti-cholinergic
Amantadine	Symmetrel	Dopaminergic
Bromocriptine	Parlodel	Dopaminergic
Carbidopa/ Levodopa	Sinemet	Dopaminergic
Entacapone	Comtan	COMT blocker
Pergolide	Permax	Dopaminergic
Selegiline	Eldepryl	MAOI

Quick Facts

- Common side effects of anti-cholinergic drugs are dry mouth and blurred vision.

H. Alzheimer's Drugs

These medications treat dementia caused by Alzheimer's disease.

Generic	Brand	Route
Tacrine	Cognex	PO
Donepezil	Aricept	PO
Rivastigmine	Exelon	PO
Galntiamine	Razadyne	PO

Quick Facts

- Vitamin E, which is an antioxidant, is usually given in combination with other drugs in the early stages of Alzheimer's disease.

I. CNS Stimulants

These medications treat narcolepsy, ADD, ADHD, and/or obesity.

Generic	Brand
Dextroamphetamine CII	Dexedrine
Methamphetamine CII	Desoxyn
Amphetamine Mixture CII	Adderall
Methylphenidate CII	Ritalin, Concerta, Metadate, Daytrana
Benzphetamine CIII	Didrex
Phendimetrazine CIII	Bontril, Plegine
Diethylpropion CIV	Tenuate
Phentermine CIV	Adipex, Fastin, Ionamin
Sibutramine CIV	Meridia
Modafinil CIV	Provigil

Quick Facts

- Daytrana is a **transdermal patch** containing methylphenidate.
- Most CNS stimulants are amphetamines.
- High potential for abuse; all of these drugs are controlled drug substances.
- All stimulants commonly cause weight loss.
- Modafinil (Provigil) – This drug is used to treat narcolepsy (excessive daytime sleepiness during normal activities).

J. Skeletal Muscle Relaxants

These medications treat muscle spasms, pain and rigidity.

Generic	Brand	Route
Baclofen	Lioresal	PO, Injection
Chlorzoxazone	Parafon Forte DSC	PO
Carisoprodol	Soma	PO
Diazepam CIV	Valium	PO, Injection
Cyclobenzaprine	Flexeril	PO
Metaxalone	Skelaxin	PO
Methocarbamol	Robaxin	PO, Injection
Orphenadrine	Norflex	PO, Injection
Tizanidine	Zanaflex	PO
Dantrolene	Dantrium	PO, Injection

CNS Questions

1. Which class of drugs is a last resort for the treatment of depression?
    a. TCA's
    b. SSRI's
    c. MAOI's
    d. SNRI's
2. Which drug has a very serious interaction with cheese and wine?
    a. Amitriptyline
    b. Phenelzine
    c. Paroxetine
    d. Trazodone
3. Which of the following drugs is a TCA (tricyclic antidepressant)?
    a. Sertraline
    b. Fluoxetine
    c. Doxepin
    d. Venlafaxine
4. Which of the following drugs is used to treat acute migaines?
    a. Citalopram
    b. Chlorpromazine
    c. Zolmitriptan
    d. Haloperidol
5. Which of the following drugs requires special pharmacy enrollment when dispensing?
    a. Risperidone
    b. Carbamazepine
    c. Sumitriptan
    d. Clozapine
6. Which of the following drugs is an anticonvulsant?
    a. Imipramine
    b. Phenytoin
    c. Alprazolam
    d. Olanzapine
7. Which of the following drugs is a benzodiazepine?
    a. Carbamazepine
    b. Thioridazine
    c. Zolpidem
    d. Diazepam
8. What controlled drug substance schedule are benzodiazepines?
    a. I
    b. II
    c. III
    d. IV
9. Which CII drug is available in a transdermal delivery system (patch)?
    a. Morphine
    b. Oxycodone
    c. Fentanyl
    d. Methadone
10. How many mg of codeine are in a Tylenol #3 tablet?
    a. 15mg
    b. 20mg
    c. 30mg
    d. 45mg

11. What controlled drug substance schedule is Tylenol#4?
  a. IV
  b. II
  c. III
  d. V
12. NSAID's should not be given to patients currently taking which of the following drugs?
  a. Acetaminophen
  b. Warfarin
  c. Valsartan
  d. Cephalexin
13. What is the mechanism of action of celebrex?
  a. ACE inhibitor
  b. Antihistamine
  c. COX-2 inhibitor
  d. Betablocker
14. Which of the following drugs is an NSAID?
  a. Ibuprofen
  b. Acetaminophen
  c. Hydrocodone
  d. Pseudoephedrine
15. Which of the following drugs treats Parkinson's disease?
  a. Furosemide
  b. Metoprolol
  c. Carbidopa/levodopa
  d. Atorvastatin
16. Which of the following drugs is not a muscle relaxant?
  a. Cyclobenzaprine
  b. Carisoprodol
  c. Tramadol
  d. Methocarbamol
17. Which of the following drugs is not an NSAID?
  a. Acetaminophen
  b. Naproxen
  c. Ibuprofen
  d. Ketoprofen

CNS Answers
1.c 2.b 3.c 4.c 5.d 6.b 7.d 8.d 9.c 10.c 11.c 12.b 13.c 14.a 15.c 16.c 17.a

IV. Gastrointestinal Drugs

A. Proton Pump Inhibitors (PPI's): suffix is *-prazole*

These medications treat gastric ulcer and esophageal reflux.

Generic	Brand	Route
Esome*prazole*	Nexium	PO, Injection
Lanso*prazole*	Prevacid	PO
Ome*prazole*	Prilosec	PO, Powder for oral suspension
Panto*prazole*	Protonix	PO, Injection
Rabe*prazole*	Aciphex	PO

Quick Facts
- PPI's work by inhibiting proton pumps from producing acid and therefore decrease the acidic environment in the stomach.
- The combination of a PPI and two antibiotics (usually Amoxil and Biaxin) are used to treat H. Pylori.

- PPI's are usually once daily dosing.
- Omeprazole (Prilosec) is the only PPI that is available over the counter (OTC).
- It may take 24 to 48 hours before these drug's effects are achieved.

B. Histamine H2 Antagonists: suffix is -tidine

These medications treat gastric ulcer and esophageal reflux.

Generic	Brand	Route
Cime*tidine*	Tagamet	PO, Injection
Rani*tidine*	Zantac	PO, Injection
Niza*tidine*	Axid	PO
Famo*tidine*	Pepcid	PO, Injection

Quick Facts
- These drugs give GI relief faster than PPI's by blocking histamine in the stomach, but long-term relief of GERD is achieved more effectively by the use of PPI's.
- All of the Histamine-2 antagonists are available OTC.

C. Antacids

These medications treat heartburn or reflux by reducing stomach acidity.

Generic	Brand	Route
Magnesium Hydroxide	Milk of Magnesia (MOM)	PO
Calcium Carbonate	Tums	PO
Magnesium Hydroxide/ Aluminum Hydroxide	Maalox	PO

Quick Facts
- Magnesium containing products may cause diarrhea.
- Aluminum containing products may cause constipation.
- Antacids can provide very rapid heartburn relief. Antacids are the best choice when immediate relief is needed.
- How to choose the appropriate acid reducing agent:
  - **Antacids** – Drug of choice for immediate relief of heartburn.
  - **H2 antagonist** – Drug of choice to take before eating something that will cause heartburn.
  - **PPI's** – Drug of choice for daily control of GERD.

D. Antidiarrheals

These medications treat diarrhea and related intestinal cramping.

Generic	Brand	Route
Diphenoxylate/Atropine (CV)	Lomotil	PO
Loperamide	Imodium	PO
Bismuth Subsalicylate (BSS)	Pepto Bismol	PO

Quick Facts
- Bismuth Subsalicylate, which an aspirin derivative, should not be given to children under 12 years old due to the possibility of the child developing Reye's syndrome.

E. Antiflatulence

These medications treat discomfort in the intestines and/or stomach due to gas.

Generic	Brand	Route
Simethicone	Mylicon, Gas-X, Phazyme	PO

Gastrointestinal Questions

1. Which of the following drugs is a Histamine-2 antagonist?
   - a. Ranitidine
   - b. Omeprazole
   - c. Diphenhydramine
   - d. Carbamazepine
2. Which of the following drugs is a proton pump inhibitor?
   - a. Trazodone
   - b. Verapamil
   - c. Metformin
   - d. Lansoprazole
3. Which antacid ingredient causes constipation?
   - a. Aluminum
   - b. Magnesium
   - c. Sodium bicarbonate
   - d. Calcium
4. Which antacid ingredient causes diarrhea?
   - a. Aluminum
   - b. Sodium bicarbonate
   - c. Calcium
   - d. Magnesium
5. Which drug should not be taken with tetracycline?
   - a. Fergon
   - b. Maalox
   - c. Centrum
   - d. None of the above should be taken with tetracycline.
6. What is the generic name for Imodium?
   - a. Lisinopril
   - b. Loperamide
   - c. Levothyroxine
   - d. Warfarin
7. Pepto Bismol should not be given to children due to the possibility of causing _____.
   - a. Chron's disease
   - b. Reye's syndrome
   - c. Serotonin syndrome
   - d. Hemophilia

Gastrointestinal Answers

1.a 2.d 3.a 4.d 5.d 6.b 7.b

V. Respiratory Drugs

A. Bronchodilator Inhalants

These medications treat asthma and bronchitis- (COPD – chronic obstructive pulmonary disease).

Generic	Brand	Action
Albuterol	Ventolin, Proventil	Beta2 agonist
Salmeterol	Serevent	Beta2 agonist
Metaproterenol	Alupent	Beta2 agonist
Pirbuterol	Maxair	Beta2 agonist
Terbutaline	Brethaire	Beta2 agonist
Epinephrine	Primatene	Alpha/Beta agonist
Ipratropium	Atrovent	Anticholinergic
Budesonide	Pulmicort	Corticosteroid
Flunisolide	Aerobid	Corticosteroid
Fluticasone	Flovent	Corticosteroid
Triamcinolone	Azmacort	Corticosteroid
Tiotropium	Spiriva	Anticholinergic
Ipratropium/Albuterol	Combivent	Anticholinergic/Beta2 agonist
Mometasone	Asmanex	Corticosteroid
Salmeterol/Fluticasone	Advair	Beta2 agonist/Corticosteroid

Quick Facts

- Albuterol is considered a "rescue inhaler" due to its rapid onset of action.
- Most asthmatic drugs are beta2 agonists, corticosteroids or a combination of both. The stimulation of beta2 receptors, which are located in the lungs, causes the relaxation of bronchial smooth muscle. This relaxation allows for easier breathing.
- Salmeterol (Serevent) - It is only used for the prevention of asthma; it will not relieve a sudden asthma attack due to its long onset of action.
- Patients should **rinse the mouth** with water after using corticosteroids to prevent oral fungal infections.

B. Oral Bronchodilator Drugs

Generic	Brand	Route
Theophylline	Theo-Dur, Slo-Bid, Uniphyll	PO
Dyphylline	Dilor, Lufyllin	PO

Quick Facts

- Theophylline (Theo-Dur, Slo-Bid) - side effects include rapid heart rate, nervousness, and nausea.
- The injectable form of Theophylline is called Aminophylline.

C. Miscellaneous Respiratory Drugs

These medications are classified as leukotriene receptor antagonists.

Generic	Brand	Route
Zafirlukast	Accolate	PO
Montelukast	Singulair	PO

Quick Facts

- Accolate and Singulair are used in the prevention and chronic treatment of asthma. Singulair is often used to treat allergy symptoms.

D. Nasal Inhalers

These medications treat allergic rhinitis.

Generic	Brand	Route
Beclomethasone	Beconase AQ	Nasal inhalation
Flunisolide	Nasarel	Nasal inhalation
Triamcinolone	Nasacort AQ	Nasal inhalation
Budesonide	Rhinocort AQ	Nasal inhalation
Fluticasone	Flonase	Nasal inhalation
Mometasone	Nasonex	Nasal inhalation

Quick Facts
- May take 1 to 2 weeks before the full benefits of these medications are achieved.

E. Antihistamines (H1 Antagonists)

These medications treat allergies such as rhinitis (runny nose) and pruritus (itching). They are also used for vertigo (balance), cough suppression, nausea, emesis (vomiting), and sleep.

Generic	Brand	Route
Brompheniramine		PO
Chlorpheniramine	ChlorTrimeton	PO
Dexchlorpheniramine		PO
Diphenhydramine	Benadryl	PO, Injection
Clemastine	Tavist	PO
Promethazine	Phenergan	PO, Injection, Suppository
Hydroxyzine	Atarax, Vistaril	PO, Injection
Azatadine	Optimine	PO
Cyproheptadine	Periactin	PO
Phenindamine	Nolahist	PO
Azelastine	Astelin	Nasal Spray
Cetirizine	Zyrtec	PO
Loratadine	Claritin	PO
Fexofenadine	Allegra	PO
Carbinoxamine	Histex	PO
Desloratadine	Clarinex	PO

Quick Facts
- Cyproheptadine (Periactin) is also used to stimulate appetite for weight gain.
- Remember, H1 antihistamines are used for allergy symptoms and H2 antihistamines are used for stomach acid suppression.

F. Decongestants

These medications treat nasal congestion. Available orally and nasally.

Generic	Brand	Route
Pseudoephedrine	Sudafed	PO
Phenylephrine	NeoSynephrine	PO, Nasal Solution
Naphazoline	Privine	Nasal Solution
Oxymeta**zoline**	Afrin	Nasal Solution
Tetrahydro**zoline**	Tyzine	Nasal Solution
Xylometa**zoline**	Otrivin	Nasal Solution

Quick Facts
- **DO NOT** use oral decongestants (pseudoephderine or phenylephrine) in patients that have severe hypertension and/or severe cardiovascular disease

55

- **DO NOT** use topical nasal decongestants for more than **3 days** due to the development of rebound congestion. Rebound congestion can be worse once the nasal decongestant is stopped.

G. Antitussives

These medications treat cough.

Generic	Brand	Class
Codeine CII		Narcotic
Dextromethorphan	Delsym	Non-Narcotic
Diphenhydramine	Diphen	Non-Narcotic
Benzonatate	Tessalon	Non-Narcotic

Quick Facts
- Do not chew or crush Benzonatate due to anesthesia (numbing) of the mouth and throat which could lead to trouble breathing.

Respiratory Questions
1. Which of the following drugs treats asthma?
   - a. Propranolol
   - b. Albuterol
   - c. Trimethoprim
   - d. Meclizine
2. Which inhaler is available over the counter?
   - a. Advair
   - b. Azmacort
   - c. Primatene
   - d. Serevent
3. Singulair is used to treat which of the following conditions?
   - a. Depression
   - b. Infection
   - c. Tachycardia
   - d. Asthma
4. Which of the following inhalers requires the patient to rinse their mouth with water after using?
   - a. Albuterol
   - b. Serevent
   - c. Combivent
   - d. Flovent
5. Which of the following antihistamines is available over the counter?
   - a. Loratadine
   - b. Fexofenadine
   - c. Cetirizine
   - d. Hydroxyzine
6. An antitussive drug treats which of the following conditions?
   - a. Depression
   - b. Allergies
   - c. Cough
   - d. Tension headaches
7. Which of the following drugs treats cough?
   - a. Benzonatate
   - b. Metoprolol
   - c. Tramadol
   - d. Temazepam

Respiratory Answers
1.b 2.c 3.d 4.d 5.a 6.c 7.a

VI. Anti-Infectives

These medications treat infections caused by bacteria or viruses.

A. Penicillins: suffix is *-cillin*

Generic	Brand	Route
Penicillin G	Bicillin LA, CR	IM, IV
Penicillin V	PenVeeK, Veetids	PO
Oxacillin		IM, IV
Cloxacillin		PO
Dicloxacillin		PO
Nafcillin	Nallpen, Unipen	IM, IV
Amoxicillin	Amoxil, Trimox	PO
Amoxicillin/Clavulanate	Augmentin	PO
Ampicillin	Principen	PO, IV
Ampicillin/Sulbactam	Unasyn	IM, IV
Piperacillin	Pipracil	IM, IV
Piperacillin/Tazobactam	Zosyn	IM, IV
Ticarcillin	Ticar	IM, IV
Ticarcillin/Clavulanate	Timentin	IV

Quick Facts

- Pregnancy category B
- Common adverse reactions include diarrhea and hypersensitivity (skin rash, itching, hives, and possibly anaphylaxis). Anaphylaxis is a potentially fatal hypersensitivity reaction, which includes severe hives and respiratory depression.
- Antibiotic induced diarrhea or the development of yeast infections can sometimes be prevented by taking a probiotic such as Lactobacillus or acidophilus.
- Amoxicillin 2gm taken 1 hour before a dental appointment is the standard regimen for the prevention of bacterial endocarditis in selected patients, such as those with heart valve replacement.

B. Cephalosporins: prefixes are *cef-* or *ceph-*

Generic	Brand	Route
Cephalexin	Keflex	PO
Cefaclor	Ceclor	PO
Cefadroxil	Duricef	PO
Cefpodoxime	Vantin	PO
Cefprozil	Cefzil	PO
Ceftibuten	Cedax	PO
Cefdinir	Omnicef	PO
Cefixime	Suprax	PO
Cefuroxime	Ceftin, Zinacef	PO, IM, IV
Cefditoren	Sprectracef	PO

Loracarbef	Lorabid	PO
*Cef*azolin	Ancef	IM, IV
*Cef*oxitin	Mefoxin	IM,IV
*Cef*triaxone	Rocephin	IM,IV
*Cef*operazone	Cefobid	IM,IV
*Cef*otaxime	Claforan	IM,IV
*Cef*tazidime	Fortaz,Tazicef	IM,IV

Quick Facts:
- Pregnancy category B
- Cephalosporins have a similar chemical structure to penicillins. Cephalosporins have a 3-7% cross-sensitivity in patients with penicillin allergies. If a person has an allergy to penicillin, then there is a small chance that they will have an allergy to cephalosporins.
- Drugs are divided into generations based on their antibacterial spectrum of activity.

C. Fluoroquinolones: suffix is -*floxacin*

Generic	Brand	Route
Cipro*floxacin*	Cipro	PO, Injection
Gati*floxacin*	Tequin	PO
Levo*floxacin*	Levaquin	PO, Injection
Moxi*floxacin*	Avelox	PO, Injection
O*floxacin*	Floxin	PO

Quick Facts
- Pregnancy category C.
- Fluoroquinolones are broad-spectrum antibacterial drugs.
- Fluoroquinolones can cause phototoxicity reactions (skin burning, redness, and rash); avoid exposure to the sun and sunlamps. Recommend sunscreen to these patients to minimize this reaction.
- Do not take any products containing calcium, iron, zinc, magnesium or dairy products within 6 hours before or 2 hours after taking fluoroquinolones due to chealation which will decrease their absorption.
- Fluoroquinolones are **contraindicated in children** (<18years) due to joint, cartilage, and tendon problems.

D. Tetracyclines: suffix is -*cycline*

Generic	Brand	Route
Tetra*cycline*	Sumycin	PO
Doxy*cycline*	Vibramycin	PO
Mino*cycline*	Minocin	PO

Quick Facts
- Pregnancy category D.
- Alternate antibiotics for patients with penicillin allergy.
- A common side effect of tetracyclines is photosensitivity.
- **Do Not** give tetracyclines to **children** due to possible **tooth discoloration**.
- Tetracyclines should **NOT** be taken with **diary products** (milk/cheese), iron, or antacids because of decreased absorption.
- Take on an empty stomach.
- Tetracycline or minocycline are used for long-term treatment and/or prevention of acne.

E. Macrolides: suffix is *–mycin* *Do NOT confuse with aminoglycosides

Generic	Brand	Route
Clarithro*mycin*	Biaxin	PO
Azithro*mycin*	Zithromax	PO, Injection
Erythro*mycin*	Ery-tab, E-mycin, EES	PO, Injection

Quick Facts
- Pregnancy category B- azithromycin, erythromycin.
- Pregnancy category C- clarithromycin.
- Macrolides are alternate antibiotics for patients with penicillin allergy.
- Clarithromycin can cause abnormal (metallic) taste.
- Azithromycin may be taken with food or on an empty stomach, but do not take with antacids.

F. Aminoglycosides: suffix is *–mycin* or *-cin*

Generic	Brand	Route
Gentami**cin**	Garamycin	Injection
Kana**mycin**	Kantrex	Injection
Tobra**mycin**	Nebcin	Injection
Amika**cin**	Amikin	Injection
Neomycin		PO
Strepto**mycin**		Injection

Quick Facts
- Almost always given IV.
- Must monitor levels due to **ototoxicity** (hearing damage) and **nephrotoxicity** (kidney damage).

G. Sulfonamides

Generic	Brand	Route
Sulfamethoxazole/Trimethoprim	Bactrim, Septra (SMZ/TMP)	PO, Injection

Quick Facts
- Pregnancy category C
- Sulfonamides are primarily used in the treatment of urinary tract infections (UTI's).
- Sulfonamides can cause phototoxicity reactions and hypersensitivity reactions.
- Patients with sulfa allergies should not take sulfonamides.
- Sulfonamides are contraindicated in nursing mothers, because sulfonamides are excreted in the milk and may cause kernicterus in the child.

H. Miscellaneous Antibiotics
1. **Vancomycin**- Given IV for severe Staphylococcus infections. Vancomycin blood levels must be monitored due to the possible development of **ototoxicity** and **nephrotoxicity**.
2. **Metronidazole (Flagyl)** - Given IV and PO. **Avoid alcohol** while taking this medication and up to 3 days after finishing the prescription to prevent the development of an Antabuse (disulfiram) type reaction. A common side effect of this medication is metallic taste.

I. Antituberculosis Drugs

These medications treat infections caused by Mycobacterium tuberculosis. They are usually given in a regimen of at least 3 drugs.

Generic	Brand	Route
Isoniazid (INH)		PO, Injection
Rifampin	Rifadin	PO, Injection
Pyrazinamide (PZA)		PO
Ethambutol	Myambutol	PO
Streptomycin		Injection

Quick Facts
- Give vitamin B6 (Pyridoxine) with Isoniazid to prevent the side effect of **peripheral neuropathy.**

J. Antiviral Drugs: suffix is –*cyclovir* or -*ciclovir*

Generic	Brand	Route
A*cyclovir*	Zovirax	PO, Injection, Topical
Fam*ciclovir*	Famvir	PO
Vala*cyclovir*	Valtrex	PO
Foscarnet	Foscavir	Injection
Gan*ciclovir*	Cytovene	PO, Injection
Valgan*ciclovir*	Valcyte	PO

K. Antifungal Drugs: suffix is -*zole*

Generic	Brand	Route
Flucytosine	Ancobon	PO
Griseofulvin	Fulvicin, Grisactin, Gris-Peg	PO
Amphotericin B	Fungizone	Injection
Nystatin	Mycostatin	PO, Topical
Ketocona*zole*	Nizoral	PO, Topical
Flucona*zole*	Diflucan	PO, Injection
Itracona*zole*	Sporanox	PO, Injection
Terbinafine	Lamisil	PO

Quick Facts
- Itraconazole (Sporanox) and Terbinafine (Lamisil) orally can be used to treat onychomycosis (nail fungus). Patients should have pretreatment liver function tests (LFT's) done due to the possibility of liver toxicity by these drugs.

L. Antimalarial Drugs: suffix is -*ine*

Generic	Brand	Route
Quin*ine*	Qualaquin	PO
Mefloqu*ine*	Lariam	PO

Chloroqu*ine*	Aralen	PO, Injection
Hydroxychloroqu*ine*	Plaquenil	PO
Primaqu*ine*		PO
Pyrimetham*ine*	Daraprim	PO
Sulfadox*ine*/Pyrimetham*ine*	Fansidar	PO
Halofantr*ine*	Halfan	PO
Atovaquone/Proguanil	Malarone	PO

M. HIV Drugs

1. Nucleoside Reverse Transcriptase Inhibitors (NRTI's)

Generic	Brand	Route
Abacavir (ABC)	Ziagen	PO
Didanosine (DDI)	Videx	PO
Emtricitabine (FTC)	Emtriva	PO
Lamivudine (3TC)	Epivir	PO
Stavudine (D4T)	Zerit	PO
Zalcitabine (DDC)	Hivid	PO
Zidovudine (AZT)	Retrovir	PO, Injection

2. Non-Nucleoside Reverse Transcriptase Inhibitors (NNRTI's)

Generic	Brand	Route
Delavirdine	Rescriptor	PO
Efavirenz	Sustiva	PO
Nevirapine	Viramune	PO

3. Protease Inhibitors (PI's)

Generic	Brand	Route
Indinavir	Crixivan	PO
Lopinavir/ Ritonavir	Kaletra	PO
Nelfinavir	Viracept	PO
Ritonavir	Norvir	PO
Saquinavir	Invirase, Fortovase	PO
Tipranavir	Aptivus	PO

4. Fusion Inhibitors

Generic	Brand	Route
Enfuvirtide	Fuzeon	Injection

<u>Quick Facts</u>
- HIV drug treatment usually consists of a regimen of multiple drug combinations.

<u>Anti-infective Questions</u>
1. Which of the following antibiotics should not be given to children?
   a. Penicillin
   b. Cephalexin
   c. Erythromycin
   d. Ciprofloxacin

2. Which of the following drugs can cause an increased risk of sunburn?
    a. Penicillin
    b. Cefuroxime
    c. Tetracycline
    d. Gentamicin
3. Which of the following antibiotics should be taken with increased water intake?
    a. Cefadroxil
    b. Azithromycin
    c. Sulfamethoxazole/trimethoprim
    d. Minocycline
4. Which auxiliary label should be attached to a prescription for metronidazole?
    a. Take with plenty of water
    b. Avoid alcohol
    c. Shake well
    d. Wash hands after using
5. Which of the following drugs is used to treat tuberculosis?
    a. Acyclovir
    b. Cefazolin
    c. Ampicillin
    d. Isoniazid
6. Which of the following drugs can cause hearing loss?
    a. Cloxacillin
    b. Vancomycin
    c. Doxycycline
    d. Cefaclor
7. Which of the following drugs is used to treat herpes?
    a. Levofloxacin
    b. Valacyclovir
    c. Tobramycin
    d. Clarithromycin
8. Which of the following drugs is used to treat yeast infections?
    a. Azithromycin
    b. Amoxicillin
    c. Fluconazole
    d. Cefprozil
9. Which of the following drugs is used to treat oral fungal infections (thrush)?
    a. Penicillin
    b. Nystatin
    c. Tetracycline
    d. Gentimicin
10. Which of the following drugs is only given by injection?
    a. Levofloxacin
    b. Erythromycin
    c. Amphotericin B
    d. Fluconazole
11. Which of the following drugs is used to treat malaria?
    a. Ciprofloxacin
    b. Mefloquine
    c. Tobramycin
    d. Ketoconazole
12. Which of the following drugs is used to treat nail fungus?
    a. Terbinafine
    b. Famciclovir
    c. Rifampin
    d. Erythromycin

13. Which of the following drugs is used to treat HIV?
    a. Zidovudine
    b. Griseofulvin
    c. Metoprolol
    d. Amitriptyline

Anti-infective Answers
1.d 2.c 3.c 4.b 5.d 6.b 7.b 8.c 9.b 10.c 11.b 12.a 13.a

VII. Ophthalmic Drugs
A. Anti-Inflammatory and/or Antibiotic Drops

Generic	Brand	Indication	Action
Flurbiprofen	Ocufen	Intraoperative miosis	NSAID
Diclofenac	Voltaren	Inflammation	NSAID
Ketorolac	Acular	Inflammation	NSAID
Fluorometholone	FML	Inflammation	Corticosteroid
Prednisolone	PredForte, Econopred	Inflammation	Corticosteroid
Dexamethasone	Maxidex	Inflammation	Corticosteroid
Rimexolone	Vexol	Inflammation	Corticosteroid
Letoprednol	Lotemax, Alrex	Inflammation	Corticosteroid
Pemirolast	Alamast	Allergic Conjuctivitis	Mast Cell Stabilizer
Nedocromil	Alocril	Allergic Conjuctivitis	Mast Cell Stabilizer
Lodoxamide	Alomide	Conjuctivitis	Mast Cell Stabilizer
Levocabastine	Livostin	Allergic Conjuctivits	Anti-Histamine
Cromolyn	Crolom	Conjuctivitis	Mast Cell Stabilizer
Ketotifen	Zaditor	Conjuctivitis	Anti-Histamine & Mast Cell Stabilizer
Tetrahydrozoline	Murine Plus	Redness, Irritation	Vasoconstrictor
Oxymetazoline	Visine	Redness	Vasoconstrictor
Naphazoline	Clear Eyes	Redness	Vasoconstrictor
Olopatadine	Patanol	Allergic Conjuctivitis	Anti-Histamine & Mast Cell Stabilizer
Emedastine	Emadine	Allergic Conjuctivitis	Anti-Histamine
Azelastine	Optivar	Allergic Conjuctivitis	Anti-Histamine & Mast Cell Stabilizer
Neomycin/Polymixin B/ Bacitracin	Neosporin	Infection	Antibiotic combination
Polymixin B/ Trimethoprim	Polytrim	Infection	Antibiotic combination
Erythromycin	Ilotycin	Infection	Antibiotic
Gentamicin	Garamycin	Infection	Antibiotic
Tobramycin	Tobrex	Infection	Antibiotic
Bacitracin	Bacitracin	Infection	Antibiotic
Ciprofloxacin	Ciloxan	Infection	Antibiotic
Gatifloxacin	Zymar	Infection	Antibiotic
Moxifloxacin	Vigamox	Infection	Antibiotic
Ofloxacin	Ocuflox	Infection	Antibiotic
Levofloxacin	Quixin	Infection	Antibiotic
Sulfacetamide	Bleph 10, Sulamyd	Infection	Antibiotic
Neomycin/Polymixin B/ Hydrocortisone	Cortisporin	Infection	Antibiotic & Cortico-steroid combination

Neomycin/PolymixinB/ Dexamethasone	Maxitrol	Infection	Antibiotic & Corticosteroid combination
Tobramycin/ Dexamethasone	Tobradex	Infection	Antibiotic & Corticosteroid combination
Sulfacetamide/ Fluorometholone	Blephamide, FML-S	Infection	Antibiotic & Corticosteroid combination

B. Glaucoma Drugs

Treats elevated intraocular pressure (ocular hypertension).

Generic	Brand	Action
Brimonidine	Alphagan, Alphagan P	Sympathomimetic
Epinephrine	Epifrin	Sympathomimetic
Dipivefrin	Propine	Sympathomimetic
Apraclonidine	Iopidine	Sympathomimetic
Carteolol	Ocupress	Betablocker
Levobunolol	Betagan	Betablocker
Betaxolol	Betoptic	Betablocker
Metipranolol	Optipranolol	Betablocker
Timolol	Timoptic	Betablocker
Pilocarpine	IsoptoCarpine	Miotic
Carbachol	IsoptoCarbachol	Miotic
Brinzolamide	Azopt	Carbonic Anhydrase Inhibitor
Dorzolamide	Trusopt	Carbonic Anhydrase Inhibitor
Bimatoprost	Lumigan	Prostaglandin Agonist
Travoprost	Travatan	Prostaglandin Agonist
Latanoprost	Xalatan	Prostaglandin Agonist

VIII. Otic Drugs

Generic	Brand	Indication	Action
Neomycin/Polymixin B/ Hydrocortisone	Cortisporin	Infection	Antibiotic & Corticosteroid combination
Ciprofloxacin/ Hydrocortisone	Cipro HC	Infection	Antibiotic & Corticosteroid combination
Benzocaine/Antipyrine	Auralgan	Pain	Anesthetic & Analgesic
Carbamide Peroxide	Debrox	Ear wax impaction	Emulsifier
Acetic Acid	Vosol, Burow's	Infection	Antibacterial
Ofloxacin	Floxin	Infection	Antibiotic

IX. Topical Drugs

A. Antihistamines

Generic	Brand	Dosage Form
Diphenhydramine	Benadryl	Cream, Lotion, Gel, Spray
Doxepin	Zonalon	Cream

B. Antibiotics

Generic	Brand	Dosage Form
Erythromycin	Emgel, Erygel,	Ointment, Gel, Solution
Gentamicin	Garamycin	Ointment, Cream
Bacitracin		Ointment
Azelaic Acid	Azelex, Finevin	Cream
Benzoyl Peroxide	Benzac, Panoxyl, Brevoxyl, Clearasil, Desquam, PersaGel, Triaz	Bar, Lotion, Gel, Cream
Clindamycin	Cleocin T	Gel, Solution, Lotion
Metronidazole	Metrocream, Metrogel, Noritate	Gel, Cream, Lotion
Mupirocin	Bactroban	Ointment, Cream
Silver Sulfadiazine	Silvadene	Cream
Clindamycin/Benzoyl Peroxide	Benzaclin	Gel
Erythromycin/Benzoyl Peroxide	Benzamycin	Gel

Quick Facts
- Azelaic Acid treats acne vulgaris.
- Metronidazole treats rosacea (remember when using Metronidazole, the patient must be counseled not to use alcohol for at least 72 hours after completing medication).
- Mupirocin treats impetigo due to Staphylococcus aureus.
- Silver Sulfadiazine treats burns (should not use this drug if patient is allergic to sulfa drugs).
- Benzoyl Peroxide can cause skin redness and peeling and is considered to be a drying agent and therefore should not be used in patients that have acne with dry skin.

C. Antifungals

Generic	Brand	Dosage Form
Butenafine	Mentax	Cream
Ciclopirox	Loprox, Penlac	Cream, Lotion, Solution
Clotrima*zole*	Lotrimin	Cream, Lotion, Solution
Econa*zole*	Spectazole	Cream
Ketocona*zole*	Nizoral	Cream, Shampoo
Micona*zole*	Monistat, Zeasorb	Cream, Ointment, Powder, Spray, Solution
Naftifine	Naftin	Cream, Gel
Nystatin	Mycostatin, Nilstat	Cream, Ointment, Powder
Oxicona*zole*	Oxistat	Cream, Lotion
Sulcona*zole*	Exelderm	Cream, Solution
Terbinafine	Lamisil	Cream, Gel
Tolnaftate	Tinactin	Cream, Solution, Gel, Powder
Undecylenic Acid	Desenex	Cream, Ointment, Powder

Quick Facts
- Penlac is a topical solution used to treat onychomycosis (nail fungus). The solution is removed from the affected nails once a week with alcohol.

D. Antivirals

Generic	Brand	Dosage Form
A*cyclovir*	Zovirax	Cream, Ointment
Pen*ciclovir*	Denavir	Cream

E. Anti-Inflammatories- (Corticosteroids): suffix is –*sone*, *-one* or *-ide*

Generic	Brand	Dosage Form
Alclometa*sone*	Aclovate	Cream, Ointment
Amcinon*ide*	Cyclocort	Cream, Ointment, Lotion
Betametha*sone*	Diprosone	Cream, Ointment, Lotion
Betametha*sone* [Augmented]	Diprolene	Cream, Ointment, Gel, Lotion
Clobetasol	Temovate	Cream, Ointment, Gel
Deson*ide*	Desowen	Cream, Ointment, Lotion
Desoximeta*sone*	Topicort	Cream, Ointment, Gel
Diflora*sone*	Psorcon E	Cream, Ointment
Fluocinol*one*	Synalar	Cream, Ointment, Solution, Shampoo
Fluocinon*ide*	Lidex	Cream, Ointment, Solution, Gel
Flurandrenol*ide*	Cordran	Cream, Ointment, Lotion, Tape
Flutica*sone*	Cutivate	Cream, Ointment
Halcinon*ide*	Halog	Cream, Ointment, Solution
Halobetasol	Ultravate	Cream, Ointment
Hydrocorti*sone*	Cortaid, Hytone, Pandel, Locoid	Cream, Ointment, Lotion, Gel, Spray
Mometa*sone*	Elocon	Cream, Ointment, Lotion
Prednicarbate	Dermatop	Cream, Ointment, Lotion
Triamcinol*one*	Kenalog, Aristocort	Cream, Ointment, Lotion

Pregnancy Categories

Category	Definition
A	Human studies show no risk in pregnancy.
B	No evidence of risk in humans, presumed safe because of animal studies.
C	Possible risk, uncertain safety, animal and human studies are lacking.
D	Positive risk, unsafe, but potential benefits may outweigh potential risks.
X	Contraindicated in pregnancy, highly unsafe.

Pregnancy Category X Drugs

- Alcohol
- Androgens
- Cocaine
- Warfarin (Coumadin)
- Diethylstilbestrol
- Penicillamine (Cuprimine)
- Isotretinoin (Accutane)
- Live vaccines (Rubella)
- "Statins"- HMG-CoA reductase inhibitors (Lipitor, etc.)
- Dutasteride (Avodart)
- Finasteride (Proscar, Propecia)
- Misoprostol (Cytotec)
- Iodides
- Thalidomide (Thalomid)

Drugs that cause Photosensitivity

Drug Category	Drug
Antihistamine/Phenothiazine	Phenergan (Promethazine)
Antibiotics	Cipro (Ciprofloxacin), Levaquin (Levofloxacin), Tetracycline, Minocycline, Doxycycline, Bactrim
Antifungals	Griseofulvin
Cardiovasculars	Thiazide diuretics (Chlorthalidone, HCTZ, Indapamide), Loop diuretics (Furosemide), Cordarone (Amiodarone)
Antipsychotics	Thorazine (Chlorpromazine)
Antiacne	Accutane (Isotretinoin)

Quick Facts

- Photosensitivity is also called phototoxicity.
- Reaction usually occurs rapidly and appears as sunburn.
- Reaction can be prevented by limiting exposure to sunlight and/or by applying sunscreens.

Drugs that Discolor the Urine

Drug	Color
Pyridium (phenazopyridine)	Red-Orange or Red-Brown
Vitamin B2 (riboflavin)	Yellow
Rifadin (rifampin)	Red or Pink
Urised (contains methylene blue)	Blue

Drugs Requiring Refrigeration

Xalatan
Abelcet
Avonex
Anectine (Succinylcholine)
Bay Hep B
Bicillin CR, LA (Penicillin G)
Byetta
Cardizem injection (Diltiazem)
Combipatch
Calcitonin injection
Desmopressin nasal (DDAVP)
Duac topical gel
Enbrel
Engerix-B
Epogen
Intron A
Lactinex

Leukeran
Ativan (Lorazepam injection)
Marinol
Methergine injection
Miacalcin nasal spray
Muse
Neupogen injection
Orapred
Foradil
Nuvaring
PEG-Intron injection
Procrit injection
Phenergan suppositories
Rebif injection
Synagis injection
Thyrolar

Insulins (Humulin/Novolin R, NPH, 70/30, U, Lantus, Humalog, Novolog)
Vaccines (DTP-diptheria, tetanus, pertussis; HepB-hepatitis; MMR-measles, mumps, rubella)

Drug Storage Temperatures

Temperature Description	Fahrenheit	Celcius
Freezer	-4 to 14 degrees	-20 to -10 degrees
Refrigerated	36 to 46 degrees	2 to 8 degrees
Cool	46 to 59 degrees	8 to 15 degrees
Room Temperature	59 to 86 degrees	15 to 30 degrees
Warm	86 to 104 degrees	30 to 40 degrees
Excess Heat	Above 104 degrees	Above 40 degrees

Vitamins

Common Name	Chemical Name	Category	Use and/or Function
Vitamin A	Retinol	Fat soluble	Eyes (retinas)/ Antioxidant
Vitamin D	Ergocalciferol	Fat soluble	Bone weakness/Rickets
Vitamin E	Tocopherol	Fat soluble	Antioxidant
Vitamin K	Phytonadione	Fat soluble	Blood clotting
Vitamin B1	Thiamine	Water soluble	Carbohydrate metabolism/Beriberi
Vitamin B2	Riboflavin	Water soluble	Mucous membranes
Vitamin B3	Niacin	Water soluble	Lipid metabolism
Vitamin B5	Pantothenic Acid	Water soluble	Metabolism/coenzyme
Vitamin B6	Pyridoxine	Water soluble	Metabolism of carbohydrates, proteins, fats
Vitamin B9	Folic Acid	Water soluble	Red blood cell production
Vitamin B12	Cyanocobalamin	Water soluble	Anemia/red blood cell production
Vitamin C	Ascorbic Acid	Water soluble	Tissue repair, collagen formation/Scurvy

Quick Facts
- Fat soluble vitamins = Vitamins A, D, E, K.
- Antioxidant vitamins = Vitamins A, C, E.
- Niacin causes red facial flushing.
- Vitamin B6 (Pyridoxine) is given in combination with Isoniazid (INH) for tuberculosis treatment.
- Vitamin B9 (Folic Acid) is given in combination with Methotrexate (MTX).
- Vitamin K (Phytonadione) can be given to an overdosed Coumadin (Warfarin) patient.
- Vitamin D (Ergocalciferol) is given with calcium supplements to increase the absorption of calcium.
- Vitamin C (Ascorbic Acid) is given with iron supplements to increase the absorption of iron.
- Vitamin E (Tocopherol) is given as an antioxidant.

Antidotes

Antidote	Poison
Acetylcycsteine (Mucomyst)	Acetaminophen (Tylenol)
Atropine	Insecticides/mushrooms
Deferoxamine	Iron
Ethanol	Ethylene glycol/methanol
Flumazenil (Romazicon)	Benzodiazepines (Valium, Xanax, etc.)
Glucagon	Hypoglycemia (excess insulin usage)
Leucovorin (Wellcovorin)	Methotrexate
Naloxone (Narcan)	Opiates (heroin, morphine, etc.)
Pralidoxime (2-PAM, Protopam)	Insecticides
Phytonadione (Vitamin K1)	Warfarin (Coumadin)
Protamine	Heparin

Dosage Forms

Buccal Tablet – A tablet that is placed between the cheek and the gum. This tablet allows for a slow release of medicine.

Capsule – A solid dosage form in which the active ingredient is inside of a gelatin shell.

Cream – A semisolid emulsion containing oil, water and usually active ingredients. Creams are not usually greasy or oily.

Effervescent Tablet – A combination of an active ingredient with sodium bicarbonate and other acids that is dissolved in water. After dissolving the tablet, the solution is then drunk.

Elixir – A water and alcohol mixture in which active ingredients are dissolved.

Emulsion – A water and oil mixture with active ingredients that must be shaken prior to use.

Enteric Coated Tablet – A tablet with a coating that allows the tablet to pass through the stomach intact and then dissolves in the intestine. This type of tablet should never be chewed or crushed.

Gel – A semisolid suspension usually containing active ingredients. They are usually in a water base. Sometimes referred to as jellies.

Lotion – A semisolid emulsion similar to creams, but they can be applied to larger areas of the body because they contain more liquid.

Lozenge – A solid dosage form that slowly dissolves in the mouth. Also known as troches.

Ointment – A greasy semisolid preparation usually containing active ingredients. They leave an oily residue on the skin.

Ophthalmic – A sterile solution, suspension or ointment containing active ingredients to be instilled or applied into the eye.

Otic – a solution or suspension containing active ingredients to be instilled into the ear.

Sublingual Tablet – A tablet that is placed under the tongue. It dissolves and is absorbed rapidly into the bloodstream.

Solution – A mixture in which one or more solid active ingredients are dissolved in liquid, usually water. The active ingredient or ingredients are uniformly dispersed throughout the mixture.

Suppository – A solid dosage form containing active ingredients that is inserted rectally or vaginally.

Suspension – A mixture in which the active ingredients are not dissolved, they are only suspended in the liquid; therefore a suspension must be shaken prior to use.

Sustained Release Tablet – A formulation of a tablet in which the active ingredient is released at a constant rate over a certain period of time. Also known as controlled release or extended release.

Syrup – A sweet concentrated solution of sugar and water in which active ingredients are added.

Tablet – A solid dosage form of different shapes and sizes. Most are to be swallowed.

Tincture – A water and alcohol mixture that has a higher alcohol concentration than elixirs.

Transdermal Patch – A drug delivery system in which the active ingredient is absorbed through the skin at a controlled rate. It is attached to the skin by adhesives.

Vaginal Tablet – A tablet that is inserted into the vagina.

CHAPTER 4

HOSPITAL PRACTICE

COMMON PHARMACY ABBREVIATIONS

How often medication is used

q	every	qh	every hour
Qd	every day	ac	before meals
Bid	twice daily	pc	after meals
Tid	three times daily	am	in the morning
Qid	four times daily	pm	in the evening
Prn	as needed	h or hr or °	hour
Q6h	every 6 hours	min	minute
Q8h	every 8 hours	ud or uad	use as directed
Q12h	every 12 hours	tat	till all taken
Hs	hour of sleep/at bedtime	d	day
Qod	every other day	AAA	apply to affected area
Stat	to be given now		

How much

Qs	Quantity sufficient	oz.	ounce
Kg	kilogram	ss	one-half
G or gm	gram	pt.	pint
mg	milligram	ml	milliliter
mcg	microgram	dl	deciliter
grn	grain	qt	quart
mEq	Milliequivilent	L	Liter
#	quantity	tsp	teaspoonful
qty	quantity	tbsp	tablespoonful
gtt	drop		

Routes of Administration

AU	each ear	SQ or SC	subcutaneous
AS	left ear	IM	intramuscular
AD	right ear	IV	intraveneous
OU	both eyes	IVP	intraveneous push
OS	left eye	ID	intradermal
OD	right eye	inj	injection
PO	by mouth	sl	sublingual
PR	per rectum	inh	inhalation
Vag	vaginally	PV	per vaginal
IVPB	intraveneous piggyback	EN	each nostril

Dosage Forms

Tab	tablet	ung	ointment
Cap	capsule	pulv	powder
Sol	solution	tinct or tr	tincture
Susp	suspension	aq	aqueous or water
Syp	syrup	gtt	drop
Supp	suppository	IU	international unit
Sol	solution	solv	solvent
Sl	sublingual	elix	elixir

Other

NPO	nothing by mouth	dx	diagnosis
NKA	no known allergy	c	with
SOB	shortness of breath	s	without
UTI	urinary tract infection	tx	therapy/ treatment
N/V	nausea and vomiting	hx	history
a	before	sx	symptom/ surgery
Syr	syringe	temp	temperature
Sig	label/directions	ha	headache
p	after	dr	delayed release
er	extended release		

Miscellaneous Drug Abbreviations

ASA – aspirin (uses: analgesic, anti-inflammatory, anti-pyretic, and anti-coagulant)
ACE inhibitor – angiotensin-converting enzyme inhibitor
APAP – acetaminophen (Tylenol- uses: analgesic, anti-pyretic)
DCN-100 - darvocet N100
EPI – epinephrine (Adrenalin- uses: bronchospasm, allergic reactions, anaphylaxis)
FA - folic acid (vitamin B9)
OTC – over the counter
NS – normal saline
Fe – iron
FeSO4 - ferrous sulfate
MgSO4 – magnesium sulfate
HCTZ – hydrochlorothiazide(diuretic)
INH – isoniazid (anti-tuberculosis)
MOM - milk of magnesia
NTG – nitroglycerin (dosage forms: sublingual, oral, aerosol, IV, ointment, patch)
PCN – penicillin
TCN – tetracycline
PNV – prenatal vitamins
MVI – multivitamin
HCL – hydrochloric acid
AIDS – acquired immunodeficiency syndrome
HIV – human immunodeficiency virus
MI – myocardial infarction (heart attack)
URI – upper respiratory infection
LRI – lower respiratory infection
HTN – hypertension
MS – multiple sclerosis
CHF – congestive heart failure
DVT – deep vein thrombosis
GERD – gastroesophageal reflux disease
Pb - phenobarabital
SMZ/TMP - sulfamethoxazole/trimethoprim (Bactrim or Septra- sulfa antibiotic)
CCB – calcium channel blocker
DDAVP – desmopressin acetate
Dig – digoxin
PCP – primary care physician
Hep – heparin (IV anti-coagulant)
D5W – 5% dextrose in water
D51/2NS – 5% dextrose and 0.45% sodium chloride
D5LR – 5% dextrose in lactated Ringer's solution

1/2NS – 0.45% sodium chloride
1/4NS – 0.2% sodium chloride
MAOI – monomamine oxidase inhibitor
KCL – potassium chloride
H_2O – water
PTU – propylthiouracil
NaCl – sodium chloride
NSAID – nonsteroidal anti-inflammatory drug
NPH – Neutral Protamine Hagedorn (intermediate acting insulin)
R – Regular insulin (rapid acting insulin)

Intravenous Solutions

Parenteral administration and aseptic technique

- Parenteral drug administration involves giving a drug via injection, which bypasses the normal defense mechanisms of the gastrointestinal tract.
- There are many different types of parenteral routes of administration. Examples include intravenous, intramuscular, subcutaneous, intra-arterial, and intradermal.
    1) Intravenous- a drug is injected directly into the vein. This route of administration has the quickest onset of action. An IV bolus injection is also known as IV push. This is when a dose of a medication is given **all at once over a short amount of time** in a relatively small dose.
    2) Intramuscular- a drug is injected directly into deep muscle mass. This route of administration can be painful. The quantity injected is usually not greater than 2.5 ml at one time. Injection sites include the upper arms and buttocks. Examples of drugs that are injected IM include antibiotics and anabolic steroids. Use 19-22 gauge 1-1.5 inch needles for IM injections.
    3) Subcutaneous- a drug is injected directly under the skin. This route of administration has a slower onset of action than intravenous. The quantity injected is usually 2 ml or less at one time. Insulin is the most common example of a subcutaneously injected drug. Use 25-31gauge and 5/16-5/8 inch needles for SC and intradermal injections.
    4) Intradermal- a drug is injected directly into the top layer of skin which will not be as deep as a subcutaneous injection. Examples of intradermal type injections include allergy tests and tuberculosis tests.
- **Aseptic technique** is the process of preparing a drug for parenteral administration. The drug will be free of both bacterial and viral contamination.
- It is extremely important to use aseptic technique when giving a drug by the parenteral route. An intravenous route of administration does NOT have any barriers of absorption and will be injected directly into the blood stream, thus bypassing the gastrointestinal tract. Therefore, the parenteral administration of drugs must be sterile and pyrogen free. Using unsterile techniques when preparing drugs could expose a patient to array of possible infections.
- There are several reasons why a drug would be given by the parenteral route:
  1) The patient does not have the capability of receiving any medication by mouth.
  2) Administering the drug directly into the blood stream allows medication to get throughout the body for a quick onset of action.
  3) The drug may not be available in an oral dosage form.
- There are benefits to giving a drug intravenously:
  1) It provides for a more rapid onset of action versus the oral route.
  2) Drugs can be given to unconscious patients.
  3) Drugs can be given to patients that have nausea and vomiting.

- **IV Infusion**- The administration of drug at a **slow and constant rate**. IV infusion could be used to give medication, rehydrate the patient or to restore nutrients or blood volume to a patient. Types of IV infusion:
    1) <u>Continuous Infusion</u>- This allows for the continuous infusion of a **large volume of fluid** over a long period of time at a constant rate.
    2) <u>Intermittent infusion</u>- This allows for a **smaller volume** to be administered over a shorter, more specific time interval.
- **Extravasation** is the leakage of injected solution from the vein into the tissue surrounding the vein.
- IV solutions should **never** be cloudy. However, TPN's can be cloudy due to the fat emulsion component.
- Multiple mixtures of medications can sometimes cause incompatibilities. These incompatibilities can usually be recognized by the presence of a milky haze, the formation of a precipitate or a change in color of the medications in the IV bag.
- IV solutions may be administered via piggyback. The benefits of piggyback administration include:
    1) Less pain for the patient because of only one venipuncture.
    2) Preventing incompatibilities from mixing multiple medicines in the same IV bag.
- IV final filters are used to remove harmful particulate matter from IV solutions. The size of **line filters** for aqueous solutions is **0.22 microns**, and 1.2 microns for larger molecule solutions such as lipids. **Particulate matter** is any undesired particles in the final solution, such as glass fragments, lint, fibers and cores.
- The most common cause of IV solution contamination is **touch** contamination. Hands should be washed thoroughly prior to sterile compounding for at least <u>30 seconds</u>.
- When washing hands, remove all jewelry and scrub hands with an antibacterial soap.
- A **filter needle** must be used when preparing medicines from ampules because small pieces of the glass ampule may fall into the IV solution when the ampule is broken open. The size of a filter needle is **5 microns.**
- **Coring** is when a needle is inserted into a rubber closure on an injectable medicine vial and a small piece of the rubber closure, the core, may be transferred into the final solution. Minimize coring by placing the bevel of the needle face upward before inserting it into a rubber closure.
- All IV solutions must be inspected for leaks, discolorations, cores, and any other particulate matter.
- IV sets are used in the administration of IV drips, IV piggybacks, continuous infusions, and intermittent infusions.
- The combination of IV medicines is affected by temperature, degree of dilution, time, and order of mixing.
- **Never** recap needles. This will prevent needle stick injuries. Always dispose of needles in a **biohazard container**, which are **red** in color.
- Inject a quantity of air **equal** to the volume of fluid withdrawn to prevent a vacuum in the injectable vial.
- Always use a syringe size that is as close as possible to the volume being measured for accuracy purposes.
- **Total Parenteral Nutrition** (TPN or Hyperalimentation) refers to large volume admixtures containing proteins, carbohydrates, and fats. TPN's are administered to patients who cannot receive their nutritional requirements orally. Aminosyn, which contains amino acids, is a typical protein drug that is used in a TPN. Dextrose is the carbohydrate supplying drug. Intralipid, which contains fats, is an example of a lipid drug used in a TPN. These large volume solutions are administered via the subclavian vein or superior vena cava because they are very hypertonic. Also added to TPN's are electrolyes, vitamins, heparin, insulin, and trace elements. A TPN is usually given over a 24 hour period.

Routes of Injectable Drugs

Route	Definition/ Use
Intradermal (ID)	Into the skin/skin tests (ex: allergies)
Subcutaneous (SC, Sub-Q)	Under the skin/insulins & vitamins
Intramuscular (IM)	Into the muscle/hormones & antibiotics
Intravenous (IV)	Into the vein/IV bolus or IV infusion
Intracardiac (IC)	Into the heart/life-threatening emergencies
Intraarterial (IA)	Into the artery
Intrathecal	Into the spinal fluid

Parts of a Syringe

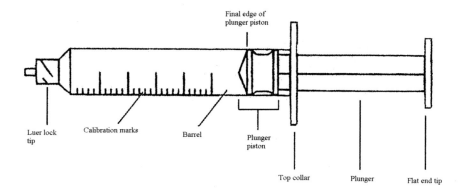

Parts of a Needle

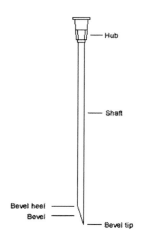

Laminar Airflow Hoods

- Laminar flow hoods are used to prepare IV solutions which require a sterile environment. These products need to be prepared in a "**Class 100**" environment which is described as containing no more than **100 particles, 5 microns or larger per cubic foot**.
- Laminar flow hoods work surfaces are made of Formica or stainless steel.
- The hoods are able to maintain a sterile environment by the use of a **HEPA (High Efficiency Particulate Air)** filter.
- The HEPA filter is the most important part of the laminar hood because it removes particles and bacteria to a **0.3 micron particle size**.
- Laminar flow hoods should be inspected and/or serviced every **6 months** or sooner, if damage is suspected, or if the hood is moved. Hood pre-filters should be cleaned or changed **every month**.
- When working inside a laminar hood:
  1) Do not wear jewelry, including watches.
  2) Do not talk or cough inside the hood.
  3) Do not place objects other than what is being prepared inside the hood.
- All work must be done at least **6 inches** inside the hood's work surface area.
- After turning on the hood, wait **30 minutes** before using it.
- Hoods should be cleaned at each shift and whenever spills occur.
- Clean hoods with **70% isopropyl alcohol** and wipe from **back to front** with a **side-to-side motion**.
- In order not to disrupt airflow, do not put larger objects at the back of the work area in front of the filter.
- Types of hoods: (Pay attention to the differences between the two types).
  1) Horizontal
  2) Vertical

Horizontal hoods

- Horizontal flow hoods are used to prepare **IV medications**.
- Air is taken in and processed through a prefilter to remove contaminents. The air then blows from the back of the hood through the HEPA filter and **across the work surface area outwards** towards the technician.
- When working in a horizontal flow hood, it is **not** necessary to wear a gown or a double set of gloves.
- Because the air is blowing towards the technician, it is pertinent that the technician not block the airflow with their hands. Therefore, the hands cannot be behind the products being worked on (i.e. vial, needle or IV bag).

Vertical hoods

- Vertical flow hoods are used to prepare **cytotoxic or hazardous drugs** such as chemotherapy medications.
- Air blows through the HEPA filter **straight down** in a vertical flow from the ceiling to the work surface area and away from the technician.
- The air in the vertical flow hood is contained and stays inside the hood. The flow hood removes any particulate matter by a special filter and the air is then recycled.
- Vertical flow hoods are generally smaller and more expensive than horizontal flow hoods.
- Vertical flow hoods are also called **biological safety hoods**.
- When working in a vertical flow hood a technician **must** wear a gown and double gloves or special chemo-gloves.
- As with the horizontal flow hoods, hands should not block the air flow that comes from above the products being worked on.

Horizontal Hood

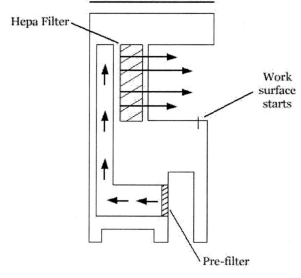

Vertical Hood

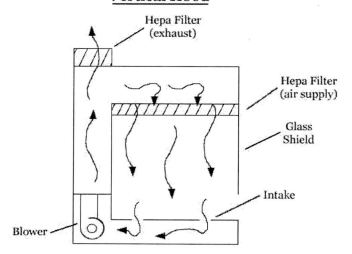

Miscellaneous

When measuring a liquid in a beaker always measure the liquid at eye level. The "meniscus" should determine the liquid point of measurement. A **meniscus** is the concave portion of a liquid inside a beaker. The higher level will be on the glass surface of the beaker and the meniscus will be the <u>lowest point</u> of the liquid. The meniscus can be seen when the liquid is viewed at eye level.

Hospital Questions

1. Which of the following statements is true regarding an IV bolus injection?
    a. Given over a long period of time
    b. Given as a large volume
    c. Given all at once
    d. Only used for TPN administration

2. Parenteral administration refers to which route of administration?
    a. Injection
    b. By mouth
    c. Inhalation
    d. Rectal

3. Which of the following routes of administration has the most rapid onset of action?
    a. Intramuscular
    b. By mouth
    c. Intravenous
    d. Rectal

4. What does the abbreviation "pc" refer to?
    a. Penicillin
    b. After meals
    c. Under the tongue
    d. By mouth

5. Which of the following statements most accurately describes intramuscular injections?
    a. Injection into the vein
    b. Injection into the epidermis
    c. Injection into the muscle
    d. Injection into adipose tissue

6. The process of sterile preparation of injectable medications in a laminar flow hood is called _____.
    a. Aseptic technique
    b. Levigation
    c. Final distillation
    d. Reconstitution

7. When disposing of used syringes, it is a good practice to recap the needles.
    a. True
    b. False

8. Which of the following dosage forms is given rectally?
    a. Tincture
    b. Sublingual
    c. Buccal
    d. Suppository

9. What does the abbreviation "ou" refer to?
    a. Both ears
    b. Right eye
    c. Left ear
    d. Both eyes

10. How many milliliters are in 1 tablespoonful?
    a. 5 ml
    b. 10 ml
    c. 15 ml
    d. 30 ml

11. Laminar airflow hoods should be turned off when not in use.
    a. True
    b. False

12. Which of the following is not a part of a syringe?
> a. Barrel
> b. Plunger
> c. Top collar
> d. Bevel

13. What is the name of the filter that maintains a sterile environment in a laminar flow hood?
> a. HEPA filter
> b. Charcoal filter
> c. Sterility filter
> d. Ozone filter

14. Which of the following needles would be used to administer an IM injection?
> a. 1/2 inch 30 gauge
> b. 1 inch 21 gauge
> c. 5/16 inch 31 gauge
> d. 1/2 inch 27 gauge

15. Which of the following solutions should be used to clean a laminar flow hood?
> a. Bleach
> b. 90% ethyl alcohol
> c. Hydrogen peroxide
> d. 70% isopropyl alcohol

16. Contamination of a final IV solution by a fragment of a rubber closure is called _____.
> a. Coring
> b. Meniscus
> c. Admixture incompatibility
> d. Precipitate

Hospital Answers

1.c 2.a 3.c 4.b 5.c 6.a 7.b 8.d 9.d 10.c 11.b 12.d 13.a 14.b 15.d 16.a

GLOSSARY

CHAPTER 5

GLOSSARY

Absorption – Occurs when a drug is transferred into the blood stream.

Auxiliary labels – Stickers on prescription bottles containing statements of warning or proper usage.

AWP – Average wholesale price (how much a product costs).

Beginning Inventory – A specific time at which merchandise is purchased.

Bioavailability – The rate and amount of a drug available at the site of action.

Brand name – The trademark name of a drug given by its maker.

Closed formulary – A policy that will only allow for the purchase of a select listing of approved drugs.

Contraindication – A condition which makes a particular treatment inadvisable.

Co-pay – The amount of a prescription that a patient with insurance must pay.

Cost of goods sold – The cost of the merchandise that will be sold.

Dispense as Written (DAW) – A request by a prescriber that the pharmacist dispense the brand name or gives the authority to the pharmacist to dispense a generic product.

Drug interaction – A situation in which a drug's effect is changed because of the addition of a second drug.

Ending inventory – What inventory is remaining after a specific time period.

FOB – Free on board; deals with transportation fees during shipping. FOB buyer means the buyer pays for delivery and shipping charges. FOB destination means the seller pays freight charges.

Generic name - Chemical name of a drug's active ingredient.

Gross profit – Profit from merchandise sold <u>before</u> expense/deductions.

Health Maintenance Organization (HMO) – A network of health care providers in which patients must stay within the network so that expenses can be more easily controlled.

Inventory – The amount of product that is not sold and on-hand at any given time.

Markdown – The amount that a product is discounted from its set price.

Markup – The difference between how much a product is purchased for and how much that product is sold for and the difference is the profit or the markup.

Material Safety Data Sheets (MSDS) – Gives instructions on handling hazardous substances.

Medicaid – A state/federal program of assistance for the poor.

Medicare – A federal program of health insurance for people over 65 years of age.

Meniscus – Used when measuring liquids in a cylinder. Always measure from the bottom of a meniscus.

Metabolism – The transformation of drugs in the body. The liver is the primary organ for drug metabolism.

NDC – Three sets of numbers that identify a manufacturer, drug, and package size. It also identifies prescription drugs approved by the FDA.

Net profit – Profit from merchandise sold after expenses/deductions.

Online adjudication – Electronic submission of prescription claims.

Open formulary – Policy that allows the purchase of any drug the doctor prescribes.

Overhead – The cost of doing business (rent, cost of goods sold, payroll and utilities).

Perpetual inventory – Inventory system that maintains a continuous record on certain items in order to always show the correct stock or count on hand; commonly seen in CII control drug substance records.

Pharmacy benefits manager (PBM) – A company whose business it is to provide drug benefit programs to insurance companies.

Piggyback – A small volume of fluid that is infused into the set of a large volume parenteral solution.

Preferred Provider Organization (PPO) – A network of health care providers in which patients may use services outside the network, but their expenses will be less if they stay within the network.

Sig – A prescriber's instructions that will be put on the prescription label.

Third party – Another party, also known as insurance, besides the patient and pharmacy that pays, to an extent, the cost of medicine.

TPN – Total parenteral nutrition; large admixtures containing dextrose, proteins, and fats. Usually also contains electrolytes, trace elements, and vitamins

Turnover rate – How often the total inventory is sold or turned over after a specific period of time.

Unit dose drug delivery system – Used in hospital and nursing home facilities; this is a system in which each patient's medicine is dispensed in individual packages.

UPC – A barcode used on items for inventory purposes.

Wholesaler – A company that receives products from manufacturers then resells those products to hospitals and pharmacies.

Worker's compensation – A type of compensation to employees that become injured while on the job.

Third Parties

There are many third parties with a wide array of plans to meet the many different needs of its customers. All third parties have one of three different types of payments: co-payment, variable rate and a percentage of the cost of the drug.

Co-payment

This type of payment charges a flat rate regardless of the cost of the medication. There is usually a set payment amount for generic drugs, brand drugs and for non-preferred drugs (a drug that is not on the insurance's formulary).

Variable rate

This type of payment will vary depending on the cost of the drug. Brand name drugs will usually have a higher payment than lower cost generic drugs.

Percentage

This plan is straight forward and charges a percentage of what a drug costs. If the drug cost is $50.00 and the percentage charge is 10%, then the charge for the drug would be $5.00 or if the drug cost is $100.00, then the payment would be $10.00.

Formulary

Hospitals try to restrict the costs of dispensing medications by developing formularies. A formulary is a list of drugs which have low cost, are safe and efficacious. A formulary limits the amount of drugs that the hospital pharmacy will carry, therefore reducing inventory and reducing the cost of doing business. The **Pharmacy and Therapeutics Committee (P&T Committee)**, which **consist of physcians, pharmacists, nurses and admininstrators, develops and maintains the formulary.** Formularies vary from hospital to hospital.

CHAPTER 6

PHARMACY CALCULATIONS

PHARMACY CALCULATIONS

Systems of Measurement

Metric System
1 mg = 1000 mcg
1 gm = 1000 mg
1 kg = 1000 gm
1 L = 1000 ml
1 dl = 100 ml

Apothecary System
1 dram = 5 ml
1 fluid ounce = 30 ml
16 fluid ounces = 480 ml = 1 pint
2 pints = 960 ml = 1 quart
4 quarts = 3840 ml = 1 gallon
1 grain = 60 mg
1/2 grain = 30 mg
1/4 grain = 15 mg

Avoirdupois System- used by manufactures
1 ounce = 30 gm
16 ounces = 454 gm = 1 pound
1 kg = 2.2 pounds

Household Measures
1/2 tsp = 2.5 ml
1 tsp = 5 ml = 1 dram
1 tbsp = 15 ml = 1/2 ounce
2 tbsp = 30 ml = 1ounce

Roman Numerals
ss - 1/2
I - 1
V - 5
X - 10
L - 50
C - 100
D - 500
M - 1000

There are several ways to solve the math problems in this section. The goal of this book is to show the simplest and most consistent ways to recognize and solve the various types of math questions presented on the PTCB exam. By keeping things consistent and simple, the equations will be easy to memorize and recognizing which equation to use in math word problems will be more manageable. This math section will be broken down into easy to understand sections. The first section is basic math review, then weight to weight, weight to volume and volume to volume, dilution, alligation, flow rates and finally business math. Kinetics and other more complicated forms of pharmacy practice calculations will not be presented in this book because those types of problems will not be on the PTCB exam.

ROMAN NUMERALS

Numbers can be expressed in different ways: **whole numbers, roman numerals, fractions, ratios, decimals, and percents.**

Examples:

1=I	20=XX	30=XXX
2=II	21=XXI	40=XL
3=III	22=XXII	50=L
4=IV	23=XXIII	60=LX
5=V	24=XXIV	70=LXX
6=VI	25=XXV	80=LXXX
7=VII	26=XXVI	90=XC
8=VIII	27=XXVII	100=C
9=IX	28=XXVIII	500=D
10=X	29=XXIX	1000=M

Let's begin with the basics and three simple rules to follow concerning roman numerals.

1) Do not use a letter more than three times.

Example: XXXX does not equal 40, XL = 40

LLLL does not equal 200, CC = 200

IIII does not equal 4, IV = 4

2) Use a larger number before a smaller number if adding.

Example: XXXV = 35

VII = 7

CLII = 152

3) Use a smaller number before a larger number if subtracting.

Example: VL = 45

CD = 400

XL = 40

Practice problems

a. 620 = _____

b. LX = _____

c. CXII = _____

d. XL = _____

e. CD = _____

f. XC = _____

g. LM = _____

h. DL = _____

i. VII = _____

j. LD = _____

k. XVII = _____

l. 900 = _____

m. 22 = _____

n. 17 = _____

o. 57 = _____

p. 30 = _____

q. 82 = _____

r. 450 = _____

Answers

a.DCXX b.60 c.112 d.40 e.400 f.90 g.950 h.550 i.7 j.450 k.17 l.CM m.XXII n.XVII o.LVII p.XXX q.LXXXII r.LD

FRACTIONS

Fractions are one whole number over another whole number to represent a portion of something. The top number is the **numerator** (which represents a portion of a whole number) and the bottom number is the **denominator** (which represents the whole number). Example: If a pie is cut in 4 pieces, and 1 piece is eaten, then the amount of pie remaining would be expressed as 3/4. The denominator represents the portion of the whole pie (4 pieces) and the numerator represents the portion of the pie that is left (3 pieces).

Proper fractions are expressed when the numerator is **smaller** than the denominator. When the numerator is divided by the denominator the answer will **ALWAYS** be a **decimal**.
> **Example:**
>> 1/1, 1/2, 2/3, 3/10
>> In the proper fraction 7/9, once 7 is divided by 9 the answer will be a decimal 0.78.

Improper fractions are expressed when the numerator is **larger** than the denominator. When the numerator is divided by the denominator the number will **ALWAYS** be a **whole number**.
> **Example:**
>> 7/2, 6/3, 8/5, 101/4
>> Also, the number 5 is the same as 5/1.
>> In the improper fraction 9/7, once the 9 is divided by the 7 the answer will be a whole number 1.29.

Always reduce fractions to the lowest common denominator.
> **Example:**
>> 4/16= 2/8 =1/4

Some numbers cannot be reduced any further e.g., 3/10, 1/2, 3/4, 2/3

Practice problems
Reduce these fractions to the lowest common denominator:

a. 8/10 = _____   b.   20/5 = _____   c.   100/60 = _____   d.   3/10 = _____
e. 6/3 = _____   f.   150/20 = _____   g.   1/6 = _____   h.   5/1 = _____
i.   15/3 = _____   j.   50/100 = _____   k.   100/50 = _____   l.   11/4 = _____

Answers
a.4/5 b.4/1 or 4 c.50/30=25/15=5/3 d.already lowest terms e.2/1 or 2 f.15/2 g.already lowest terms h.5 i.5/1 or 5 j.1/2 k.2/1 or 2 l.already lowest terms

Mixed Fractions are a combination of whole numbers and fractions.
> **Example:**
>> 2 3/4

To convert a mixed fraction into a fraction, multiply the whole number by the denominator (2 x 4 = 8), then add the numerator to the sum of the whole number and denominator (8 + 3 = 11). Place the sum (11) over the denominator from the mixed fraction (11/4). This can now be converted into a decimal by dividing the numerator by the denominator which equals 2.75 (the improper fraction 11/4, the whole number 2.75, and 2 3/4 are all equal and mean the same thing). To take this one step further, if there is a problem requiring the multiplication of a whole number (8) by a mixed fraction (6 2/3), conversion to a proper fraction is necessary. First, convert the whole number to a fraction (8 is the same as 8/1) then convert the mixed fraction to an improper fraction (6 2/3 equals 20/3). Now set up the equation and multiply.

$$\frac{8}{1} \times \frac{20}{3} = \frac{160}{3}$$

Practice Problems
a. 8 2/3 = _____   b.   2 6/7 = _____   c.   12 6/10 = _____

Answers
a.8.6[8x3=24,24+2=26;26/3=8.6] b.2.85[2x7=14;14+6=20;20/7=2.85] c.12.6[12x10=120;120+6=126;126/10=12.6]

RATIOS

Ratios are fractions in a different format. A ratio is the comparison of two things expressed in numbers "this is to that as that is to this" and is commonly expressed as a number with a colon then another number (the fraction 2/3 can be expressed as a ratio 2:3).

Example:

1:1, 1:2, 2:3, 3:10, 7:2, 6:3

- Both fractions and ratios represent parts of a number that when divided will give a whole number or a decimal.

    Example:

    An Epi-pen is represented in a ratio of 1:1000. This means that there is 1 part epinephrine per 1000 parts of solution. If written in a fraction it would be written as 1/1000. When the numerator is divided by the denominator it will give a number expressed as a decimal (because it is a proper fraction). This decimal (0.001) represents the concentration of epinephrine in the solution.

- The example that will be used throughout this math section will be the dilution of household bleach for cleaning. A bleach solution of 1 part bleach to 9 parts water in a fraction would be expressed as 1/10 and if expressed as a ratio would be 1:10.

- It is important to be able to convert fractions/ratios to whole numbers or decimals. This is easily done by dividing the numerator by the denominator.

    Remember:

    - If the **smaller** number is the numerator the final answer will be a **decimal**.
    - If the **larger** number is the numerator the final answer will be a **whole number**.

    Example:

2/4 = 0.5	10/20 = 5/10 = 0.5
4/2 = 2	16/4 = 8/2 = 4/1 = 4
3/4 = 0.75	24/3 = 8/1 = 8

Practice Problems

a. 3/10 = _____
b. 10/2 = _____
c. 8/16 = _____
d. 16/8 = _____
e. 8/3 = _____
f. 9/14 = _____
g. 14/9 = _____
h. 3/4 = _____
i. 9/3 = _____
j. 20/6 = _____
k. 100/50 = _____
l. 50/100 = _____
m. 2/8 = _____
n. 162/43 = _____
o. 87/114 = _____
p. 3/8 = _____

Answers

a. 0.3 b. 5 c. 0.5 d. 2 e. 2.67 f. 0.64 g. 1.56 h. 0.75 i. 3 j. 3.33 k. 2 l. 0.5 m. 0.25 n. 3.76 o. 0.76 p. 0.375

DECIMALS

Decimals are expressed in 10th, 100th, 1000th and beyond in a decimal form. It is **very important** to understand how a decimal is expressed, placed and what the numerical value of the decimal means. For example: 0.5 = 5/10, 0.05 = 5/100, 0.005 = 5/1000, the decimal 0.5 is ten times larger than 0.05 which can make the difference between life and death when dosing a patient (0.5 x 10 = 5 vs. 0.05 x 10 = 0.5). Both fractions and ratios can easily be converted into decimals by dividing the first number by the second number for ratios and by dividing the numerator by the denominator for fractions.

> **Example:**
>> Let's solve for a decimal with the fraction of 1/2 and ratio 1:2. On the calculator push the number 1 (numerator) and divide by the number 2 (denominator) which will give the decimal 0.5.

- When **adding or subtracting** decimals, it is **crucial** to line up and add up the decimal points correctly.
  > **Example:**
  >> 0.086 + 0.125 + 3.126
  >>
  >> Set up as follows: 0.086
  >> 0.125
  >> + 3.125
  >> 3.337

Practice Problems

1) 88.6	2) 3.75	3) 83.7
+ 6.25	+ 0.67	+ 0.006

Answers
1) 94.85 2) 4.42 3) 83.706

- When **multiplying** decimals, add up the numbers **after** decimal points and move the decimal point to the left that many times in the final answer. In the example (3.**126** x 1.**86** there are a total of 5 numbers **after** the decimal points) move the decimal point to the left five times in the final answer. The answer is 5.81436 not 5814.36 or 581.436.

> **Example:**
>> 3.**126**   (3 decimal points behind the whole number)
>> x1.**86**   (2 decimal points behind the whole number)
>> 5.**81436** (5 decimal points behind the whole number)

Practice Problems

1) 23.7	2) 167	3) 14.87
x 0.6	x 2.6	x 0.087

Answers
1) 14.22 2) 434.2 3) 1.29369

Important note:

If a 0 is placed at the end of 0.75 to make the decimal 0.750 the significance of the number has not changed. Five more zeros could be added to express the decimal 0.75000000 and the number still equals 0.75. If a 0 is placed in front of 0.75 the concentration will completely change. The new number or strength 0.075 is 10 times less than 0.75.

Practice Problems
Which number is larger?

1)	0.64 or 0.085	2)	1.24 or 0.25	3)	0.25 or 0.125
4)	0.87 or 0.62	5)	0.005 or 0.06	6)	0.001 or 0.002

Answers
1) 0.64 2) 1.24 3) 0.25 4) 0.87 5) 0.06 6) 0.002

PROPORTIONS

Proportions express the equality between two ratios or fractions. **Most** pharmacy calculations are ratio/proportion problems that can be solved by using simple cross multiplication. Ratios and fractions consist of two numbers that relate to each other and can be expressed several ways.

Example: 2 mg per 10 ml means
$$\frac{2\ mg}{10\ ml}$$

2mg:10 ml means
$$\frac{2mg}{10\ ml}$$

2 mg is dissolved in 10 ml means
$$\frac{2\ mg}{10\ ml}$$

10 ml contains 2 mg means
$$\frac{2mg}{10\ ml}$$

Important Note:

On the certification exam, only a few equations will be needed to solve MOST of the math problems encountered. The most difficult part of math word problems is deciding which equation to use, how to manipulate that equation to solve the problem and then having the correct placement of the numbers to achieve the correct answer. Once this is done, it becomes simple math. To keep things simple, a brief description is given below describing the various word problems encountered on the exam. The example of adding water to bleach will be used to demonstrate how to apply the different equations.

Cross Multiplication

- Cross multiplication will be used in **MOST** of the word problems encountered on the PTCB exam. It is very important to remember that in cross multiplication everything **must be** proportionally equal (A/B **MUST** equal C/D). For example, a proportion question would be phrased as such: if diluting 1 part bleach with 10 parts water how many parts of bleach would be needed in a 150 parts of water to maintain the **same** concentration.
- Cross multiplication will be used when doing conversions, business math, weight to weight, weight to volume and volume to volume problems.

Dilution

- Dilution involes reducing something of a higher strength to make a product of lower strength. For example, household bleach can be diluted by adding a diluent like water to make a weaker, less concentrated and more useable form of bleach for cleaning.
- In dilution problems, cross multiplication **cannot** be used because the new, weaker, concentration is not proportionally equal to the original concentration.

Alligation

- Alligation involves mixing a solution of a high concentration with a solution of a lower concentration to make a solution with a concentration somewhere between the two original solutions. For example, mixing 1 part bleach to10 parts water to a solution of 5 parts bleach to 10 parts water will give a new concentration somewhere **between** the two concentrations. The new concentration **cannot and will not** be higher or lower than the original concentrations.

CROSS MULTIPLICATION
Ratio (A/B = C/D) and Proportion A:B = C:D

Cross multiplication is an extremely important equation to understand when solving pharmacy calculations, so let's explain it step-by-step. With many pharmacy calculation problems, there are several ways to solve for "X." For consistency and simplification, cross multiplication will be used to solve ratio and proportion problems throughout the rest of this review.

- When using the equation A/B = C/D, it is very important to understand that A/B is **ALWAYS** equal to C/D and C/D is **ALWAYS** equal to A/B. To explain further, 1/2 is proportionally equal to 5/10 and 3/4 is proportionally equal to 75/100 but 1/2 is **NOT** proportionally equal to 3/4. A glass half-empty is proportionally equal to a glass half-full. A glass half-full is **not** proportionally equal to a glass three-fourths full. When two equations or statements are proportionally equal cross multiplication can be used to solve for "X".
  Example:
    If 4 balls cost $7.00 how much would 3 balls cost?
    Fraction: 4 balls/$7.00 = 3 balls/$X
    Ratio: 4:7 = 3:X
- It is called cross multiplication because the numerator on the left side of the equation is being cross multiplied with the denominator on the right side of the equation and the denominator on the left side of the equation is being cross multiplied with the numerator on the right side of the equation. Remember, solve for "X" by isolating it.
- The first and most important thing to do is to set up the equation correctly. For consistency, always place what is known on the left side of the equation and what is being solved for ("X") on the right side of the equation.
- It is known that 4 balls cost $7.00. Set this up in a fraction form.
  4 balls
  $7.00
- Now, on the right side of the equation solve for "X" (what is not known). How much does 3 balls cost?
  4 balls = 3 balls
  $7.00   X
- It is <u>very important</u> to line the units up correctly or the answer will be wrong. Balls are the numerator and the cost of balls is the denominator. "X" could be placed anywhere in the equation and solved for as long as the units line up correctly and three of the four things are known.
- Now, let's change the fraction to multiplication by cross multiplying and isolating "$X". Multiply 4 balls by "X" and 3 balls by $7.00.
  3 balls x $7.00 = 4 balls x X
- Continue to isolate "X" by moving 4 balls to the other side of the equation and divide to solve for "X".
  3 balls x $7.00 = X x ~~4 balls~~
   4 balls   ~~4 balls~~
  3 ~~balls~~ x $7.00 = X
   4 ~~balls~~
  $21 = X
   4
  $5.25 = X
- So, 4 balls cost $7.00 and 3 balls cost $5.25. "X" could be placed anywhere in the equation and solved for as long as three of four things are known and what is being solved for are proportionally equal things. As in the problem just solved, 4 balls costing $7.00 and 3 balls costing $5.25 are proportionally equal.
  7/4 = X/3
  7 x 3 = X x 4
  (7 x 3)/4 = X
  21/4 = X
  5.25 = X (3 balls cost $5.25)

Practice Problems

1. If 6 candy bars cost $10.00, how much would 2 candy bars cost?

6 candy bars = 2 candy bars
$10.00   X

2 candy bars x $10 = 6 candy bars x X

(2 candy bars x $10)/ 6 candy bars = X

$20/6 = X

$3.33 = X

2. Digoxin is available in a concentration of 0.3mg per 2 ml. How many milliliters are required to administer 30 mg?

Convert to a fraction and cross multiply.

0.3 mg = 30 mg
2 ml   X

2 ml x 30 mg = 0.3 mg x X

60 ml x mg = 0.3 mg x X

60 ml x mg = X
 0.3 mg

60 ml x ~~mg~~ = X
 0.3 ~~mg~~

200 ml = X

3. Amphotericin B is available in a concentration of 100 mg/20 ml. What quantity is required for a 3 mg dose?

100 mg = 3 mg
20 ml   X

3 mg x 20 ml = 100 mg x X

60 mg x ml = 100 mg x X

60 mg x ml = X
 100 mg

60 ~~mg~~ x ml = X
 100 ~~mg~~

0.6 ml = X

4. How much Ceclor 250 mg per 5 ml suspension should be dispensed for a 350 mg dose?

250 mg = 350 mg
 5 ml   X

350 mg x 5 ml = 250 mg x X

1750 mg x ml = 250 mg x X

1750 ~~mg~~ x ml = X
 250 ~~mg~~

7 ml = X

5. What volume of a 100 mg/ml injectable should be drawn to prepare a 120 mg dose?

100 mg = 120 mg
1 ml   X

1ml x 120 mg = 100 mg x X

120 ml x mg = 100 mg x X

120 ml x ~~mg~~ = X
 100 ~~mg~~

1.2 ml = X

6. What volume (ml) of digoxin 1.0 mg per 4 ml injection will deliver a dose of 0.12 mg?

$\dfrac{1.0 \text{ mg}}{4 \text{ ml}} = \dfrac{0.12 \text{ mg}}{X}$

4 ml x 0.12 mg = 1 mg x X

0.48 ml x mg = 1 mg x X

$\dfrac{0.48 \text{ ml x } \cancel{mg}}{1 \cancel{mg}} = X$

0.48 ml = X

7. A doctor orders Augmentin 250mg. Augmentin 150 mg per 5 ml is the only strength that the pharmacy has in stock. How many milliliters will be needed to administer a 250mg dose?

$\dfrac{150 \text{ mg}}{5 \text{ ml}} = \dfrac{250 \text{ mg}}{X}$

5 ml x 250 mg = 150 mg x X

1250 ml x mg = 150 mg x X

$\dfrac{1250 \text{ ml x } \cancel{mg}}{150 \cancel{mg}} = X$

8.33 ml = X

PERCENTS (%)

Percent is an expression of a number per hundredths. It explains how much of something there is per 100 parts of that something. For example, if there are 100 puzzle pieces and 25 of them are black, then it should be said that 25% of the puzzle pieces are black or 25 out of 100 puzzle pieces are black. To express a decimal as a percent multiply by 100 or move the decimal two places to the right.

Example:

> If 5 apples out of 100 are bad, what percent are bad?
> **Fraction:** 5/100 (5 apples per 100 apples are bad)
> **Ratio:** 5:100 (5 apples in 100 apples are bad)

- To convert a fraction or a ratio to a decimal, divide 5 by 100 (5/100 = 0.05).
- To convert a decimal to a percent, multiply the decimal by 100 and add a percent sign (0.05 x 100 = 5 %).

It can be said that:

Percent: 5%   5% of apples are bad
Fraction: 5/100 5 apples per 100 are bad
Decimal: 0.05   5 apples in 100 are bad
Ratio: 5:100 5 apples in 100 are bad

Example

> If 35 apples out of 157 are rotten, what percent are rotten?
> Set up the equation and cross multiply. Look at it this way, if 35 apples out of 157 apples are bad, how many or what percent of 100 apples would be bad?
>
> $$\frac{35}{157} = \frac{X}{100}$$
> $$35 \times 100 = 157 \times X$$
> $$3500 = 157 \times X$$
> $$\frac{3500}{157} = 22.3\%$$

Example:

> If there are 120 apples and 27 are lost, what percent of the apples are remaining?
> $$120 - 27 = 93$$
> There are 93 good apples out of 120 total apples remaining. Do not get confused. If the question were asking what percent of apples are lost, the fraction would be 27/120, but the question is asking what percent remains. 93 out of 120 remain, so, in a fraction form, it would be set up as 93/120 remain.
>
> $$\frac{93}{120} = \frac{X}{100}$$
> $$93 \times 100 = 120 \times X$$
> $$9300 = 120 \times X$$
> $$\frac{9300}{120} = X$$
> $$77.5\% = X$$

Practice percent to decimal conversion:

1. What is 10% of 60?
    10/100 = 0.1
    0.1 x 60 = 6
2. What is 5% of 80?
    5/100 = 0.05
    0.05 x 80 = 4
3. What is 10% of 90?
    10/100 = 0.1
    0.1 x 90 = 9

CONVERSIONS

- There will be many conversion questions on the exam. It is extremely important to memorize the conversion table on page 82. For example, it is necessary to remember that 1 kg = 2.2 lbs.
  Example:
  If a person weighs 84 lbs, what is the patient's weight in kg?
- Cross multiplication, as explained previously, will be used in these types of proportion problems. Solve for "X" by placing what is known on the left (1 kg = 2.2 lbs) and what is being solved for (what is not known) on the right (84 lbs = X Kg).
  $$\frac{1 \text{ kg}}{2.2 \text{ lbs}} = \frac{X}{84 \text{ lbs}}$$
- Remember, **ALWAYS** line up the units correctly. In this example, the numerator is expressed in kg on the left side, so the numerator **must** also be expressed in kg on the right side. Furthermore, since the denominator is expressed in lbs on the left side, then the denominator must also be expressed in lbs on the right side.
  $$\frac{1 \text{ kg}}{2.2 \text{ lb}} = \frac{X \text{ kg}}{84 \text{ lb}}$$

  1 kg x 84 lb = 2.2 lb x X

  $$\frac{84 \text{ kg x } \cancel{lb}}{2.2 \cancel{lb}} = \frac{2.2 \cancel{lb} \text{ x X}}{2.2 \cancel{lb}}$$

  38.18 kg = X
- There will be questions asking to convert many different units of measure, especially the conversion of grams (gm) to milligrams (mg) to micrograms (mcg). Knowing how to express the unit of measure as a decimal (10ths, 100th and 1000th) is important in this type of conversion.
  1 kg = 1000 gm
  1 g = 1000 mg
  1 mg = 1000 mcg

- **Or if going from kg to gm to mg to mcg multiply** by 1000 at each step:
  Kg (multiply by 1000)→ gm x 1000 → mg x 1000 → mcg
  Liters L x 1000→ ml

- If going from mcg to mg to gm to kg divide by 1000 at each step:
  Kg ← (divide by 1000) ← gm /1000 ← mg /1000← mcg
  Liters L /1000 ←ml
  Example:
  A 1 gm tablet can be expressed in mg, mcg or kg by moving the decimal point over three places to the left or to the right, or by multiplying or dividing by 1000 depending on the direction of conversion for each unit of measure.
    - When converting large units of measure to smaller units of measure multiply by 1000.
      Example:
      Convert 5 gm to mg
      5 x 1000 = X
      5000 mg = X
    - If converting smaller units of measure to a larger unit of measure divide by 1000.
      Example:
      Convert 5 mg to gm
      5/1000 = X
      0.005 gm = X

Convert:

1. Convert 2.5 oz to grams.

- Set up the equation, line up the units, cross multiply and solve for "X". Put what is **known** on the left side (1 oz = 28.4 gm), remember conversions will not be given, they will have to be memorized. What is **not known** goes on the right side, how many "X gm" are in 2.5 oz?

$$\frac{1 \text{ oz}}{28.4 \text{ gm}} = \frac{2.5 \text{ oz}}{X}$$

28.4 gm x 2.5 oz = 1 oz x X

$$\frac{71 \text{ gm x } \cancel{oz}}{1 \cancel{oz}} = \frac{1 \cancel{oz} \text{ x X}}{1 \cancel{oz}}$$

71 gm = X

Practice Problems

1. Convert 10 grams to mg.
   To convert gm to mg multiply by 1000 or move the decimal over to the right three spaces.
   10 gm x 1000 = 10,000 mg

2. Convert 15 drams to ml.
   1 dram = 5 ml
   $$\frac{5ml}{1 \text{ dram}} = \frac{X \text{ ml}}{15 \text{ dram}}$$
   5ml x 15 dram = 1 dram x X
   75 = 1 x X
   75 ml = X

3. Convert 10 mg to grains.
   Depending on the reference used, 1 grain can be between 60 to 65 mg. In this book we will use 60mg = 1 grain.
   $$\frac{1 \text{ gr}}{60 \text{ mg}} = \frac{X \text{ gr}}{10 \text{ mg}}$$
   1 gr x 10 mg = 60 mg x X
   10 = 60 x X
   $$\frac{10}{60} = X$$
   0.166 gr = X

4. Convert 5 gallons to ml.
   1 gallon = 3840 ml
   $$\frac{3840 \text{ ml}}{1 \text{ gallon}} = \frac{X \text{ ml}}{5 \text{ gallon}}$$
   3840 ml x 5 gallon = 1 gallon x X
   19200 ml = X

5. Convert 5 tablespoons to ml.
   1 tablespoon = 15 ml
   $$\frac{15 \text{ ml}}{1 \text{ tbsp}} = \frac{X \text{ ml}}{5 \text{ tbsp}}$$
   15 ml x 5 tbsp = 1 tbsp x X ml
   75 ml = X

6. Convert 3 pints to ml.
   1 pt = 480 ml
   480 ml = X ml
    1 pt   3 pt
   480 ml x 3 pt = 1 pt x X ml
   1440 ml = X

7. 3 & 1/2 teaspoons are equivalent to how many ml?
   1 tsp = 5 ml
   5 ml = X ml
   1 tsp   3.5 tsp
   5 ml x 3.5 tsp = 1 tsp x X
   17.5 ml = X

Practice Problems
1) Express the fraction 6/10 as a ratio.
2) Express 6/10 or 6:10 as a decimal.
3) Express 0.6 as a percent.
4) Convert 60% to decimal form.
5) Convert 60% to a fraction or decimal.

Answers
1)6:10 2) divide 6 by10 which equals 0.6 3)multiply by 100 which equal 60% 4) divide by 100 which equals 0.6 5) convert 60/100 to the lowest denominator $\underline{60} = \underline{6} = \underline{3} = 0.6$
100   10   5

Convert:

Decimal	Ratio	Fraction	Percent
1) 0.75	_____	_____	_____
2) _____	_____	_____	80%
3) _____	6:1000	_____	_____
4) 0.25	_____	_____	_____
5) _____	_____	9/15	_____
6) _____	_____	_____	33%

Answers

Decimal	Ratio	Fraction	Percent
1) 0.75	3:4	3/4	75%
2) 0.8	8:10	8/10 or 4/5	80%
3) 0.006	6:1000	6/1000 or 3/500	0.6%
4) 0.25	2:8	2/8 or 1/4	25%
5) 0.6	9:15	9/15	60%
6) 0.33	3:9	3/9 or 1/3	33%

Convert to kg, gm, mg, mcg, L and ml:
1. 150 mg + 3 gm = _____
2. 3 kg + 8 gm = _____
3. 0.675 mg + 23.75 mg = _____
4. 0.625 gm + 8.2 mg = _____
5. 8.65 ml + 3.67 L = _____

Convert:

	kg	gm	mg	mcg
1)	_____	8 gm	_____	_____
2)	_____	_____	0.375 mg	_____
3)	_____	0.0067	_____	_____
4)	_____	_____	872 mg	_____
5)	_____	_____	_____	2006 mcg
6)	24 kg	_____	_____	_____

	gallon	liter	pint	oz	tbsp	tsp
7)	1 gal	_____	_____	_____	_____	_____
8)	_____	_____	1 pt	_____	_____	_____
9)	_____	10 L	_____	_____	_____	_____
10)	_____	_____	_____	16 oz	_____	_____
11)	_____	_____	_____	_____	_____	1 tsp
12)	_____	0.5 L	_____	_____	_____	_____
13)	_____	_____	_____	_____	3 tbsp	_____

Conversion Problems

1. How many oz. are in 1 gallon?
2. How many ml are in 1 gallon?
3. How many qt. are in 1 gallon?
4. How many gallons are in 9000 ml?
5. How many pt. are in 9000 ml?
6. How many oz. are in 3 L?

PTCB TYPE CONVERSION PROBLEMS:

Example:

1. Nitrostat 1/150 grain is equal to how many milligrams?

      a.   0.2 mg
      b.   0.4 mg
      c.   0.5 mg
      d.   0.1 mg

Remember, this is a fraction, which is the same as the ratio 1:150, which can be converted to a decimal by dividing 1 into 150. 1/150 = 0.007 gr

From the systems of measurement chart: 1 gr = 60 mg

$$\frac{1\ gr}{60mg} = \frac{0.007\ gr}{X}$$

60 mg x 0.007 gr = 1 gr x X

$$\frac{0.42\ mg\ x\ \cancel{gr}}{1\ \cancel{gr}} = \frac{1\ \cancel{gr}\ x\ X}{1\ \cancel{gr}}$$

0.42 mg = X

Practice Problems

1. Nitrostat 1/300 grain is equivalent to how many milligrams?

$$\frac{1}{300} = 0.003\ gr$$

1 gr = 60 mg

$$\frac{1\ gr}{60\ mg} = \frac{0.003\ gr}{X}$$

60 mg x 0.003 gr = 1 gr x X

$$\frac{0.18\ mg\ x\ \cancel{gr}}{1\ \cancel{gr}} = \frac{1\ \cancel{gr}\ x\ X}{1\ \cancel{gr}}$$

0.18 mg = X

2. Nitrostat 1/30 mg is equivalent to how many grains?

$$\frac{1}{30} = 0.033\ mg$$

$$\frac{60\ mg}{1\ gr} = \frac{0.033mg}{X}$$

1 gr x 0.033 mg = 60 mg x X

$$\frac{0.033\ gr\ x\ \cancel{mg}}{60\ \cancel{mg}} = \frac{60\ \cancel{mg}\ x\ X}{60\ \cancel{mg}}$$

0.00055 gr = X

3. How many gallons are in 100 pints?

8 pt = 1 gallon

$$\frac{8\ pt}{1\ gal} = \frac{100\ pt}{X}$$

100 pt x 1 gal = 8 pt x X

$$\frac{100\ \cancel{pt}\ x\ gal}{8\ \cancel{pt}} = \frac{8\ \cancel{pt}\ x\ X}{8\ \cancel{pt}}$$

12.5 gal = X

4. How many liters are contained in 110 pints?
   1 pt = 480 ml
   1 liter = 1000ml
   480 ml x 110 pt = 52800 ml

   $\dfrac{1 \text{ liter}}{1000 \text{ ml}} = \dfrac{X}{52800 \text{ ml}}$

   1 liter x 52800 ml = 1000 ml x X

   $\dfrac{52800 \text{ liter x } \cancel{ml}}{1000 \cancel{ml}} = \dfrac{1000 \cancel{ml} \text{ x X}}{1000 \cancel{ml}}$

   52.8 liter = X

5. How many quarts are contained in 12,300 ml?
   1 quart = 960 ml

   $\dfrac{1 \text{ qt}}{960 \text{ ml}} = \dfrac{X}{12300 \text{ ml}}$

   12300 ml x 1 qt = 960 ml x X

   $\dfrac{12300 \cancel{ml} \text{ x qt}}{960 \cancel{ml}} = \dfrac{960 \cancel{ml} \text{ x X}}{960 \cancel{ml}}$

   12.81 qt = X

6. 105 ml is equivalent to how many fluid ounces?
   1 oz = 30 ml

   $\dfrac{1 \text{ oz}}{30 \text{ ml}} = \dfrac{X}{105 \text{ ml}}$

   105 ml x 1 oz = 30 ml x X

   $\dfrac{105 \cancel{ml} \text{ x oz}}{30 \cancel{ml}} = \dfrac{30 \cancel{ml} \text{ x X}}{30 \cancel{ml}}$

   3.5 oz = X

7. 150 grams is equivalent to how many mg?
   Multiply by 1000 or move to the right three spaces
   150 $\cancel{gm}$ x $\dfrac{1000 \text{ mg}}{1 \cancel{gm}}$ = 150,000 mg

8. 105 mg is equivalent to how many grams?
   Divide by 1000 or move to the left three spaces
   105 $\cancel{mg}$ x $\dfrac{1 \text{ gm}}{1000 \cancel{mg}}$ = 0.105 gm

9. 15 tablespoon is equivalent to how many ml?
   1tbsp =15 ml
   15 tbsp = X ml
   15 $\cancel{tbsp}$ x $\dfrac{15 \text{ ml}}{1 \cancel{tbsp}}$ = 225 ml

10. How many gallons of betadine solution would be needed to repackage 100 pints?
    1 gallon = 8 pints
    100 $\cancel{pt}$ x $\dfrac{1 \text{ gal}}{8 \cancel{pt}}$ = 12.5 gal

11. How many 200 mg doses are contained in 5 grams of cephalexin?
    Convert 5 gm to mg by multiplying 5 gm by 1000 or move the decimal to the right by three spaces.
    5 gm x 1000 = 5000 mg
    $\dfrac{5000 \cancel{mg}}{200 \cancel{mg}}$ = 25 doses

12. How many 150 mg doses are contained in 10 gm of cephalexin?
   Convert 10 gm to mg
   Multiply 10 gm x 1000 = 10,000 mg
   $\dfrac{10,000 \text{ mg}}{150 \text{ mg}}$ = 66.7 doses

13. What is the total weight if 0.5 gm is added to 50 mcg?
   Convert 0.5 gm to mcg.
   Multiply 0.5 gm x 1000 = 500 mg x 1000 = 500,000 mcg
   50 mcg + 500,000 = 500,050 mcg
   Divide by 1000 to get mg
   $\dfrac{500,050}{1000}$ = 500.05 mg

14. What is the total weight if 0.03 gm is added to 500 gm?
   0.03 gm + 500 gm = 500.03 gm

Weight/Weight, Weight/Volume, and Volume/Volume

- **The denominator will tell the dosage form and the numerator is the weight or volume of the substance.** These problems are easily solved by using cross multiplication which can be expressed as a percentage or in units of measure, such as volume (ml) or weight (gm, mg, etc.).

Weight/Weight (W/W):

- **W/W** will **always** be expressed in **gm/gm, kg/kg, mg/mg, mcg/mcg** or number of parts per 100 parts. W/W is a proportional cross multiplication problem that involves one substance of weight being compounded with another substance of weight. The big difference between W/W and W/V or V/V is that in W/W calculations, both substances, the drug (numerator) and the diluent (denominator), are solids or semisolids that can be weighed.

Example:

Compounding 60% Kenalog (drug) in ointment (diluent) would contain 60 gm (numerator) of kenalog per 100 gm (denominator) of ointment. 60% = 60 **gm** per 100 **gm** of ointment. Make sure to keep the units correct.

Question:

What would be the _**weight**_ of Kenalog in 140 gm of a 60% kenalog ointment?

- This question asks if there are 60 gm (60 %) of a drug in 100 gm of diluent (ointment) how many grams of the drug would be in 140 gm of diluent. This question is dealing with proportions so use cross multiplication.
- The most difficult aspect to these types of questions is deciding where the "X" goes. Since 140 gm of ointment is the diluent, 140 gm is the denominator. The numerator is "X" which is the percent or the amount drug in grams (the amount of drug that are in 140 gm of diluent). Think of it like this, if there are 60 gm (60%) of a drug in 100 gm of ointment then proportionally speaking 84 gm of the same drug will be in 140 gm of ointment.

$$\frac{60 \text{ gm}}{100 \text{ gm}} = \frac{X \text{ gm}}{140 \text{ gm}}$$

$$60 \times 140 = 100 \times X$$

$$8400 = 100 \times X$$

$$\frac{8400}{100} = X$$

$$84 \text{ gm} = X$$

The question can be turned around to ask:

What would be the _**percent strength**_ of Kenalog ointment if 140 gm of ointment contains 84 gm of Kenalog?

$$\frac{X \text{ gm}}{100 \text{ gm}} = \frac{84 \text{ gm}}{140 \text{ gm}}$$

$$84 \times 100 = 140 \times X$$

$$8400 = 140 \times X$$

$$\frac{8400}{140} = X$$

$$X = 60\%$$

- The only difference between the "**weight**" question and the "**percent strength**" question is the placement of the "X". The percent strength question is asking if there are 84 gm of Kenalog in 140 gm of diluent, what would be the percent strength or amount (in grams) in 100 gm of diluent?

Question: *be careful when answering this question.*

What would the ***percent strength*** of Kenalog ointment be if 140 gm of ointment is added to 84 gm of kenalog?

- This question is asking something a little different. The concentration in the previous question was 84 gm **in** 140 gm of diluent. This question is asking to add 84 gm **to** 140 gm of diluent. In the previous question the total amount of drug and diluent was 140 gm. Now 84 gm is being added to 140 gm so the new total amount of drug would be 224 gm.

$$\frac{X\ gm}{100\ gm} = \frac{84\ gm}{224\ gm}$$

100 x 84 = 224 x X

8400 = 224 x X

$\frac{8400}{224}$ = X

37.5% = X

Question:

What amount of 60% Kenalog would be in one pound of ointment?

If 60 gm (60%) of the drug is in 100 gm of diluent how much drug would be in one pound? Cross multiply and solve for "X".

1 lb = 454 gm

$$\frac{60\ gm}{100\ gm} = \frac{X\ gm}{454\ gm}$$

60 x 454 = 100 x X

27240 = 100 x X

$\frac{27240}{100}$ = X

272 gm = X

Weight/Volume (W/V):

- **W/V** will **always** be expressed in **grams/milliliters**. The numerator will **always** be expressed in **grams** and the denominator will **always** be expressed in **milliliters**. Weight to volume consists of adding a **substance (in grams)** such as NaCl into a **liquid diluent** such as water.

  Example:

  Normal Saline contains 0.9% (which is 0.9 grams) of sodium chloride in 100 ml of water. What *percent* would be in 80 ml of water?

  $\dfrac{0.9 \text{ gm}}{100 \text{ ml}} = \dfrac{X \text{ gm}}{80 \text{ ml}}$

  0.9 x 80 = 100 x X

  72 = 100 x X

  $\dfrac{72}{100} = X$

  0.72% = X

  The question could also ask:

  What would be the *weight* (how many grams) of NaCl that would be in 80 ml of water of a 0.9% NaCl solution?

  $\dfrac{0.9 \text{ gm}}{100 \text{ ml}} = \dfrac{X \text{ gm}}{80 \text{ ml}}$

  0.9 x 80 = 100 x X

  72 = 100 x X

  $\dfrac{72}{100} = X$

  0.72 gm = X

  Question:

  If there is 0.72 gm in 80 ml of solution, how many **mg** would be in 80 ml of solution?

  - Since there is 0.72 gm in 80 ml and the question is asking how many mg are in 80 ml. Gm will need to be changed to mg.

  Answer: 0.72 x 1000 = 720mg

  Question:

  What would be the **percent** of NaCl in one tablespoonful of a 80 ml solution?

  - Be careful when answering this question because the percent strength does not change. If all 80 ml of the solution are used or just 15 ml of the solution is used, the concentration will still remain the same. The percent strength **only** changes when the concentration of the solution changes.

  Answer: 0.72%

  Example:

  How many mg of Drug A would it take to make a pint of 1:10,000 solution?

  Remember a W/V problem will always be expressed as gm/ml.

  $\dfrac{1 \text{ gm}}{10,000 \text{ ml}} = \dfrac{X}{480 \text{ ml}}$

  1 x 480 = 10,000 x X

  $\dfrac{1 \times 480}{10,000} = X$

  $\dfrac{480}{10,000} = X$

  0.048 gm = X

  48 mg = X

Volume/Volume (V/V):

- **V/V** will usually be expressed in **milliliters/milliliters** (liquid preparations), but can also be expressed in pints/pints, gallons/gallons, liters/liters, etc. Both the drug and the diluent are liquid preparations.

Example:

In V/V equations, 70% alcohol would be expressed as 70 ml/100 ml. (70 ml of isopropyl alcohol is contained in 100 ml of solution).

How much isopropyl alcohol would be contained in 183 ml of a 70% isopropyl alcohol solution?

$$\frac{70 \text{ ml}}{100 \text{ ml}} = \frac{X \text{ ml}}{183 \text{ ml}}$$

$70 \times 183 = 100 \times X$

$12,810 = 100 \times X$

$\dfrac{12,810}{100} = X$

$128.1 \text{ ml} = X$

Example:

What would be the percent strength of isopropyl alcohol if 183 ml of diluent contains 128.1 ml of isopropyl alcohol?

$$\frac{X}{100 \text{ ml}} = \frac{128.1 \text{ ml}}{183 \text{ ml}}$$

$100 \times 128.1 = 183 \times X$

$12,810 = 183 \times X$

$\dfrac{12,810}{183} = X$

$70\% = X$

DILUTION

Dilution problems involve diluting (or reducing) the strength of a stock solution to a lower strength. An example of dilution would be mixing water with bleach to make a usable cleaning solution. Remember, W/W, W/V and V/V are all proportionately equal equations but dilution proplems are **not** proportionally equal because the percent strength is changed.

FORMULA: **(Q1) (S1%) = (Q2) (S2%)**
Q1 stands for **quantity** on the left side of the equation (**original** starting quanity or volume).
Q2 stands for **quantity** on the right side of the equation (**final** quantity or volume).

S1 stands for **strength** on the left side of the equation (**starting percent concentration** of original solution).
S2 stands for **strength** on the right side of the equation (**percent concentration** of final diluted solution).

- This is **not** cross multiplication because the original volume is not proportionately equal to the final diluted volume. Like cross multiplication there will be three known "things" and one unknown, "X", that will need to be solved for. The dilution formula is used to solve for a new diluted quanity in a final solution or a new percent strength in a diluted final solution. As always, make sure to keep the units lined up correctly.

Question:
If there is a 10% stock solution, but what is needed is 200 ml of a 4% solution, how much diluent will need to be added? It is **VERY IMPORTANT** to recognize what the question is asking for, so that the right equation will be used. The question is asking to **reduce** a concentrate by diluting a stock solution of higher concentration, with a diluent like water (or any other diluent), to make a less concentrated solution. Remember, **do not** use cross multiplication, A/B **does not equal** C/D in dilution problems.

- Remember, just as in W/W, W/V, or V/V, when a percent of an original volume is given the percent amount will be placed over 100 ml or mg. For example, a 10% stock solution means 10 ml/100 ml or 10 gm/100 ml. The percent can either be converted to a decimal before solving for "X" or the percentages can be left as is. For consistency percentages will be converted to decimals.
  (Q1) (S1%) = (Q2) (S2%)
  Q1 = 200 ml
  Q2 = X
  S1 = 4% or 0.04
  S2 = 10% or 0.1

  (200)(0.04) = (X)(0.1)
  8 = (X)(0.1)
  $\frac{8}{0.1}$ = X
  80 = X

- It is **extremely important** to understand what this answer means. What is wanted is a **total** of 200 ml of a 4% solution. So, 80 ml of the 10% stock solution must be used to make this diluted solution. 120 ml of diluent would be added to make a total of 200 ml of a final 4% solution. Realize, 80 ml will be subtracted from the total 200 ml (200 ml – 80 ml = 120 ml of diluent) to determine how much diluent will need to be added to the 80 ml used to make a final concentration of a 4% solution in 200 ml.

Dilution Problems: (Q1) (S1%) = (Q2) (S2%)

1. How many grams of a 1.5% hydrocortisone cream can be made from 280 grams of 2.5% cream?
   - First convert the percent to a decimal.
     2.5/100 = 0.025
     1.5/100 = 0.015

   - Now set up the equation and solve for "X". Put what is known on the left side. If there are 2.5 % (2.5 gm/100 gm) in 280 gm how many grams are needed to make a 1.5 % (1.5 gm/100 gm) hydrocortisone cream compound?
     Set up the equation.
     Q1 is 280 gm
     Q2 is X
     S1 is 0.025 gm
     S2 is 0.015 gm

     280 gm x 0.025 gm = X gm x 0.015 gm
     7 gm = X gm x 0.015 gm
     $\dfrac{7\ gm}{0.015\ gm}$ = X
     466.7 gm = X

2. How many ml of a 1:100 stock solution must be used to prepare 200 ml of a 1:500 solution?
   - Remember a ratio is the same as a fraction and can easily be set up in decimal form. Set the problem up the same way the previous problem was set up. Convert the stock solution to a decimal and set up the equation to solve for "X".
     Q1 = 200 ml
     Q2 = X
     S1 = 1/500 = 0.002
     S2 = X
     Q1S2 = Q2S2
     0.002 x 200 ml = 0.01 x X
     0.4 ml = 0.01 x X
     0.4 ml/0.01 = X
     40 ml = X

Practice Problems

1. How many grams of a 2% hydrocortisone cream can be made from 350 grams of 4% cream?
     S1 = 4/100 = 0.04
     S2 = 2/100 = 0.02
     Q1 = 350 gm
     Q2 = X
     0.04 x 350 gm = 0.02 x X
     14 gm = 0.02 x X
     14 gm/0.02 = X
     700 gm = X

2. How many grams of a 1% hydrocortisone cream can be made from 350 grams of 2% cream?

S1 = 2/100 = 0.02
S2 = 1/100 = 0.01
Q1 = 350 gm
Q2 = X
0.02 x 350 gm = 0.01 x X
7 gm = 0.01 x X
7 gm/0.01 = X
700 gm = X

3. How many ml of a 1:50 stock solution must be used to prepare 150 ml of a 1:250 solution?

S1 = 1:250 = 1/250 = 0.004
S2 = 1:50 = 0.02
Q1 = 150 ml
Q2 = X
0.004 x 150 ml = 0.02 x X
0.6 ml = 0.02 x X
0.6 ml/0.02 = X
30 ml = X

4. How many 20 mg minoxidil tablets would be needed to make 100 ml of a 10% solution?

- Remember this is a w/v problem so 10% is the same as 10 gm/100 ml. Make sure the units match up because there is a tablet (solid) mg and a solution gm/ml.

S1 = 10% = 10 gm/100 ml. Since the answer is in mg change 10 gm to mg by either moving the decimal over to the right three spaces or multiply by 1000.
(10 x 1000 = 10,000 mg/100 ml)
S1 = 10,000 mg
Q1 = 100 ml
Q2 = X
S2 = 20 mg
Q1 x S1 = Q2 x S2
100 ml x 10,000 mg/100 ml = X x 20 mg
1,000,000 ml x mg/100 ml = X x 20 mg
10,000 mg = X x 20 mg
10,000 mg/20 mg = X
500 tablets = X

5. How many 100 mg minoxidil tablets would be needed to make 1/2 liter of a 10% solution?

Convert 10% to gm = 10 gm/100 ml = 10,000 mg/100 ml
Convert 1/2 liter to ml = 1/2 liter = 500 ml
S1 = 10,000 mg/100 ml
Q1 = 1/2 liter = 500 ml
S2 = 100 mg
Q2 = X
Q1 x S1 = Q2 x S2
500 ml x 10,000 mg/100 ml = X x 100 mg
50,000 mg = X x 100 mg
500 tablets = X

109

6. How many 100 mg Clindamycin capsules are required to compound the following prescription: Clindamycin 3.5%, Propolene glycol 5%, Isopropyl alcohol qs 500 ml?

- Always extract whatever is needed from the problem. The question is specifically asking for Clindamycin. Propylene glycol and isopropyl alcohol are not needed, ignore them.

Convert 3.5% to gm = 3.5 gm/100 ml, then convert to mg which is the unit of the final answer.

3.5 gm/100 ml to mg by multiplying by 1000. (3.5 gm x 1000 =3500 mg/100 ml).

$Q1 \times S1 = Q2 \times S2$

$Q1 = X$

$Q2 = 500$ ml

$S1 = 100$ mg

$S2 = 3500$ mg/100 ml

$X \times 100$ mg $= 500$ ml $\times 3500$ mg/100 ml

$X \times 100$ mg $= 1,750,000$ mg $\times$ ~~ml~~/100 ~~ml~~

$X \times 100$ mg $= 17,500$ mg

$X = \dfrac{17,500 \text{ ~~mg~~}}{100 \text{ ~~mg~~}}$

$X = 175$ capsules

7. A 20 ml dose of a mixture prescribed for pain relief contains 10mg morphine, 10mg cocaine, 5 ml alcohol, 5 ml cherry syrup qs with water. How many 30 mg morphine sulfate tablets are needed to prepare 480 ml of the solution?

- Remember to extract only the information needed.

$Q1 = 480$ ml

$Q2 = X$

$S1 = 10$ mg/20 ml

$S2 = 30$ mg

$Q1 \times S1 = Q2 \times S2$

480 ml $\times 10$ mg/20 ml $= X \times 30$ mg

$\dfrac{4800 \text{ ~~ml~~} \times \text{mg}}{20 \text{ ~~ml~~}} = X \times 30$ mg

240 mg $= X \times 30$ mg

$\dfrac{240 \text{ ~~mg~~}}{30 \text{ ~~mg~~}} = X$

8 tablets $= X$

ALLIGATION

Alligation is the process of taking a substance of high concentration and mixing it with a substance of lower concentration to achieve a desired concentration in a specific volume. Notice, an alligation question will give two specific concentrations and ask how much of each will be needed to achieve the desired concentration at a specific volume. For example, how much 70% alcohol must be mixed with 10% alcohol to make 480 ml of a 50% alcohol solution?

- It is **extremely important** to recognize that alligation problems are very different from dilution problems. Remember, **dilution** is reducing the strength of a high concentrate with a diluent to make a lower concentrate. **Alligation** is mixing a high concentrate with a low concentrate to make a solution of a concentrate that will be in the **middle** of the two original concentrates.

In the above example, the 70% alcohol is the high concentrate and the 10% is the low concentrate. How much of each solution will be needed to make a final concentration of 50%?

- To solve alligation problems, use the **"tic-tac-toe"** method.

Tic-Tac-Toe:
- Put the two concentrations given on the left side (70% and 10%). Place the **higher concentration on the top** and the **lower concentration on the bottom** and **the desired concentration in the middle.**

70%		
	50%	
10%		

- Now subtract diagonally, 70 – 50 = 20, place the 20 at the bottom right hand side. Now, subtract 50 - 10 = 40, place the 40 at the top right hand side.

70%		**40 parts**
	50%	+
10%		**20 parts**

- Now, solve by adding the right column 40 + 20 = 60. The number 60 is the total parts made once 40 parts of a 70% solution are mixed with 20 parts of a 10% solution. The compound made by this mixture is 60 total parts of a 50% concentrate.

70%		40 parts
	50%	+
10%		20 parts
		60 total

- Now, solve for how many ml's of each concentrate it would take to make 480 ml of a 50% concentrate. Take the volume of each concentration given (40 parts of 70% and 20 parts of 10%), divide by 60 and multiply by the final volume desired which is 480 ml.
  40/60 x 480ml = 320 ml
- A total of 320 ml of the 70% concentrate is needed to make 480 ml of a 50% concentration.
  20/60 x 480 ml = 160 ml
- A total of 160 ml of the 10% concentrate is needed to make 480 ml of a 50% concentration.
- As a final check make sure the ml of each mixture total 480 ml.
  320 ml + 160 ml = 480 ml of a 50% solution.

Practice Problems

1. How much of 50% alcohol must be mixed with 20% alcohol to make 1000 ml of a 35% alcohol solution ?

```
50              15
        35      +
20              15
                30
```

15/30 x 1000 ml = 500 ml
15/30 x 1000 ml = 500 ml
Check: 500 ml + 500 ml = 1000 ml

2. How much of 100% alcohol must be mixed with 50% alcohol to make 1/2 liter of a 70% alcohol solution?
- Remember 1 liter = 1000 ml.
    1/2 liter = 500 ml

```
100             20
        70      +
50              30
                50
```

For 100% solution: 20/50 x 500 ml = 200 ml
For 50% solution: 30/50 x 500 ml = 300 ml
Check: 200 ml + 300 ml = 500 ml

3. How much of 70% ethanol must be mixed with 40% ethanol to make 1 pint of 50% ethanol solution?
    1 pt = 480 ml

```
70              10
        50      +
40              20
                30
```

For 70% solution: 10/30 x 480ml = 160 ml
For 40% solution: 20/30 x 480ml = 320 ml
Check: 160ml + 320ml = 480 ml

4. How much of D90W must be mixed with D40W to make 1 pint of D50W solution?
- Remember D90W is 90% dextrose in water, D50W is 50% dextrose in water and D40W is 40% dextrose in water.
    1 pint = 480 ml

```
90              10
        50      +
40              40
                50
```

For 90% solution: 10/50 x 480 ml = 96 ml
For 40% solution: 40/50 x 480 ml = 384 ml
Check: 96 ml + 384 ml = 480 ml

5. How many ml of 70% Dextrose should be mixed with water to make 360 ml of 25% Dextrose solution?

$$
\begin{array}{ccc}
70 & & 25 \\
 & 25 & + \\
0 & & \underline{45} \\
 & & 70
\end{array}
$$

For 70% solution: 25/70 x 360 ml = 129 ml
For 0% solution: 45/70 x 360ml = 231 ml
Check: 129 ml + 231 ml = 360 ml

6. Thirty grams of 8.5% zinc oxide ointment is prescribed by a dermatologist. The pharmacy has 10% zinc oxide ointment and aquaphor available in stock. How many grams of each will be required to compound this prescription?

Remember aquaphor is 0%

$$
\begin{array}{ccc}
10 & & 8.5 \\
 & 8.5 & + \\
0 & & \underline{1.5} \\
 & & 10
\end{array}
$$

For 10% ointment: 8.5/10 x 30 gm = 25.5 gm
For 0% ointment: 1.5/10 x 30 gm = 4.5 gm
Check: 25.5 gm + 4.5 gm = 30 gm

FLOW RATES

FLOW RATE = Drops per minute = <u>Volume</u> x Drop factor
Time

OR

<u>Volume (ml)</u>   x   <u>Drop factor (gtts)</u> = <u>X gtts</u>
Time (minutes)   Volume (ml)   min

OR

<u>gtt</u> = <u>gtt</u>
ml   ml

1. A patient with sepsis has an order for Kefzol 1 gm in 50 ml of D5W IVPB over 30 minutes. The drip factor is 40 gtts/ml. How many gtt/minute should be given?

- The hardest part to flow rate problems is separating the information given and placing the correct information into the equation. The patient is going to receive 1 gm or 50 ml over a 30 minute period of time. The question is asking how many drops per minute will the patient receive. If there are 40 gtts/ml and the patient needs 50 ml (40 gtts/ml x 50 ml = 2000 gtts) then a total of 2000 gtts will be given over a 30 minute period of time. Now, the only information needed is how many drops per minute will be given over 30 minutes. Divide 2000 gtts/30 min = 67 gtts/min.

    Formula: <u>volume (ml)</u>   x   <u>drop factor (gtts)</u> = X <u>gtts</u>
    time(minutes)   volume (ml)   min

    <u>50 ml</u>   x <u>40 gtts</u> = X
    30 min   ml
    <u>2000 ml</u> x gtts = X
    30 min x ml
    <u>67 gtts</u> = X
    min

2. What is the flow rate of an IV if 125 ml of a drug is to be infused over 2 hours? The administration set delivers 60 gtts/ml.

    2 hours = 120 minutes
    <u>125 ml</u> x <u>60gtts</u> = X
    120 min   ml
    <u>7500 ml</u> x gtts   = X
    120 min x ml
    <u>63 gtts</u> = X
    min

3. What is the flow rate of an IVPB containing 150 ml of gentamicin? The solution is to be infused over a 1 hour period and the administration set is calibrated to deliver 10 drops per ml.

    <u>150 ml</u> x <u>10 gtts</u> = X
    60 min   ml
    <u>1500 ml</u> x gtts = X
    60 min x ml
    <u>25 gtts</u> = X
    min

4. What is the flow rate of an IVPB containing 200 ml of metronidazole? The solution is to be infused over a 5 hour period and the administration set is calibrated to deliver 5 drops per ml.

$$\frac{200 \text{ ml}}{300 \text{ min}} \times \frac{5 \text{ gtts}}{\text{ml}} = X$$

$$\frac{1000 \text{ ml} \times \text{gtts}}{300 \text{ min} \times \text{ml}} = X$$

$$\frac{3 \text{ gtts}}{\text{min}} = X$$

5. What is the flow rate of an IVPB containing 110 ml of clindamycin? The solution is to be infused over a 30 minute period and the administration set is calibrated to deliver 55 drops per ml.

$$\frac{110 \text{ ml}}{30 \text{ min}} \times \frac{55 \text{ gtts}}{\text{ml}} = X$$

$$\frac{6050 \text{ ml} \times \text{gtts}}{30 \text{ min} \times \text{ml}} = X$$

$$\frac{202 \text{ gtts}}{\text{min}} = X$$

Flow Rates using Proportions:

1. An infusion order is received for Vancomycin 750 mg in 1500 ml of D10W. The Vancomycin is to be infused at a rate of 15 mg/hr. What would be the flow rate in ml/hr?

- Look at the question. Determine what is given and what variable needs to be solved. There is 750 mg in 1500 ml to be infused at a rate of 15 mg/hr. Line up the units and cross multiply.

$$\frac{750 \text{ mg}}{1500 \text{ ml}} = \frac{15 \text{ mg/hr}}{X \text{ ml}}$$

15 mg/hr x 1500 ml = 750 mg x X

22,500 mg/hr x ml = 750 mg x X

$$\frac{22,500 \text{ mg/hr} \times \text{ml}}{750 \text{ mg}} = X$$

30 ml/hr = X

2. An infusion order is received for Rocephin 2 gm in 500 ml of D10W. The Rocephin is to be infused at a rate of 50 mg/hr. What would be the flow rate in ml/hr?

- Do not forget to convert gm to mg so that the units match. Change 2 gm to mg by multiplying 2 gm x 1000 = 2000 mg.

$$\frac{2000 \text{ mg}}{500 \text{ ml}} = \frac{50 \text{ mg/hr}}{X \text{ ml}}$$

500 ml x 50 mg/hr = 2000 mg x X

25,000 ml x mg/hr = 2000 mg x X

$$\frac{25,000 \text{ ml} \times \text{mg/hr}}{2000 \text{ mg}} = X$$

12.5 ml/hr = X

3. The physician orders 500 ml of iron dextran to be infused over 20 hours. How many ml/hr should the IV pump be programmed for?

$$\frac{500 \text{ ml}}{20 \text{ hr}} = \frac{25 \text{ml}}{\text{hr}}$$

4. The physician orders 750 ml of Lactated Ringers solution to be infused over 24 hours. How many ml/min should the IV pump be programmed for?

- Do not forget to change from hours to minutes by multiplying by 60 minutes.

$$\frac{750 \text{ ml}}{24 \text{ hr}} = \frac{31.25 \text{ ml}}{\text{hr}}$$

- If 31.25 ml are infused in one hour how many ml are infused every minute?

1 hr = 60 min

$$\frac{31.25 \text{ ml}}{\text{hr}} \times \frac{1 \text{ hr}}{60 \text{ min}} = X \text{ ml/ min}$$

$$\frac{31.25 \text{ ml}}{60 \text{ min}} = X$$

$$\frac{0.52 \text{ ml}}{\text{min}} = X$$

Business Math

The good news in this business math section is that there are no new equations to learn. The trick to solving these problems, like all the other math sections, is setting the equation up correctly.

Cost:
- When solving for the cost of a drug, use simple cross multiplication and solve for "X".

Example:

A 250 tablet bottle of ferrous sulfate costs $15.30, what would be the cost of 50 tablets?

- Set up equation and cross multiply.

$$\frac{250 \text{ tablets}}{\$15.30} = \frac{50 \text{ tablets}}{X}$$

$15.30 x 50 tablets = 250 tablets x X
$765 x tablets = 250 tablets x X
$$\frac{\$765 \text{ tablets}}{250 \text{ tablets}} = X$$
$3.06 = X

Practice Problems

1. A 400 tablet bottle of ferrous sulfate cost $11.70. What would be the cost of 50 tablets?

$$\frac{\$11.70}{400 \text{ tablets}} = \frac{X}{50}$$

$11.70 x 50 tablets = 400 tablets x X
$585 x tablets = 400 tablets x X
$$\frac{\$585 \text{ tablets}}{400 \text{ tablets}} = X$$
$1.46 = X

2. A 600 tablet bottle of Ibuprofen cost $ 105.00. What would be the cost of 150 tablets?

$$\frac{\$105.00}{600 \text{ tablets}} = \frac{X}{150 \text{ tablets}}$$

$105 x 150 tablets = 600 tablets x X
$15,750 x tablets = 600 tablets x X
$$\frac{\$15{,}750 \text{ x tablets}}{600 \text{ tablets}} = X$$
$26.25 = X

3. A 350 tablet bottle of Gemfibrozil cost $9.50. What would be the cost of 35 tablets?

$$\frac{\$9.50}{350 \text{tablets}} = \frac{X}{35 \text{ tablets}}$$

$9.50 x 35 tablets = 350 tablets x X
$332.50 x tablets = 350 tablets x X
$$\frac{\$332.50 \text{ tablets}}{350 \text{ tablets}} = X$$
$0.95 = X

Markup:

- Markup is the difference between what a pharmacy pays for a product and what a pharmacy sells a product for (retail price).

Markup = Selling Price – Purchase price

Or

Markup + Cost = Selling Price

Example:

The markup for a $40.00 vial of antibiotic is 20%. What is the retail price for this medicine?

- First convert percent to decimal.

$\dfrac{20\%}{100} = X$

$0.20 = X$

- Now, figure out how much, in dollars, is 20% of $40.00. This is done by multiplying the decimal form of 20% (0.20) by $40.00

$40.00 x 0.20 = X

$8.00 = X

$8.00 is 20% of $40.00 so add the $8.00 to $40.00 to get the retail price.

$40.00 + $8.00 = $48.00

Example:

Drug A cost $50.00 per 100 tablets. After markup, Drug A is sold for $89.00. What is the markup of Drug A?

$89.00 - $50.00 = $39.00 markup

Practice Problems

1. The markup for a $50.05 vial of antibiotic is 10%. What would be the retail price for this medication?

$50.05 x 0.10 = $5.01

$50.05 + $5.01 = $55.06

2. The markup for a $60.99 vial of antibiotic is 15%. What would be the retail price for this medication?

$60.99 x 0.15 = $9.15

$60.99 + $9.15 = $70.14

3. The cost of 350 tablets of ibuprofen 600 mg is $70.99. If the pharmacy marks up the cost by 5%, what would the retail charge for 100 tablets be?

- First figure out what the new cost of 350 tablets would be.

$70.99 x 0.05% = $3.55

$70.99 + $3.55 = $74.54 is the new cost of 350 tablets.

- Now figure out what the cost of 100 tablets would be.

$\dfrac{\$74.54}{350\ tablets} = \dfrac{X}{100\ tablets}$

$74.54 x 100 tablets = 350 tablets x X

$7454.00 x tablets = 350 tablets x X

$\dfrac{\$7454.00\ tablets}{350\ tablets} = X$

$21.30 = X

4. The cost of 250 tablets of ibuprofen 200 mg is $9.50. If a pharmacy markups the cost by 15% and adds $3.00 dispensing fee, what would be the retail charge for 120 tablets?

$9.50 x 0.15 = $1.43
$9.50 + $1.43 = $10.92

$$\frac{\$10.92}{250 \text{ tablets}} = \frac{X}{120 \text{ tablets}}$$

$10.92 x 120 tablets = 250 tablets x X
$1310.40 x tablets = 250 tablets x X
$$\frac{\$1310.40 \text{ tablets}}{250 \text{ tablets}} = X$$
$5.24 = X
$5.24 + $3.00 (dispensing fee) = $8.24

5. If the AWP for a bottle of 50 Percodan is $60.99 with a 15% markup and a $6.50 dispensing fee is charged, what would be the retail price for 45 tablets?

$60.99 x 0.15 = $9.15
$60.99 + $9.15 = $70.14

$$\frac{\$70.14}{50} = \frac{X}{45}$$

$70.14 x 45 = 50 x X
$3156.30 = 50 x X
$$\frac{\$3156.30}{50} = X$$
$63.13 = X
$63.13 + $6.50 = $69.63

Discount:

- Discounts are usually given to expedite the sale of slow moving merchandise or to attract customers to drive sales.

Discount = Markup – Markdown

Example:

    The AWP for a drug is normally $46.99 but comes with a 20% discount from the wholesaler. What would be the cost of this drug?

- **Remember when converting a percent to a decimal divide by 100, then multiply the decimal by the AWP of the drug.**

$$\frac{20}{100} = 0.2$$

$46.99 x 0.2 = $9.40
So 20% of $46.99 is $9.40 so subtract $9.40 from $46.99.
$46.99 - $9.40 = $37.59

Practice Problems

1. The AWP for a drug is $30.99 with a 10% discount from the wholesaler. What would be the cost of this drug?

$$\frac{10}{100} = 0.10$$

$30.99 x 0.10 = $3.10
$30.99 - $3.10 = $27.89

2. The AWP for a drug is $36.99 with a 15% discount from the wholesaler. What would be the cost of this drug?

$$\frac{15}{100} = 0.15$$

$36.99 x 0.15 = $5.55

$36.99 - $5.55 = $31.44

3. If the cash discount on a $500.00 wholesaler invoice is $50.00, what is the percent discount for this invoice?

If $500.00 is 100%, what percent is $50.00? Set up the equation and cross multiply.

$$\frac{100\%}{\$500} = \frac{X}{\$50}$$

100% x $50 = $500 x X

5000% x $ = $500 x X

$$\frac{5000\% \text{ x } \$}{-\$500} = \frac{\cancel{\$500} \text{ x } X}{\cancel{\$500}}$$

10% = X

Markup Rate:

Selling Price – Purchase Price = Markup

Markup is the amount above the cost of merchandise purchased that a product is sold for (also known as the gross profit).

Example:

If a toy is purchased for $5.00 and sold for $6.00 the markup is $1.00 (the **gross profit** is $1.00, but the **net profit** is what is left of the $1.00 once all other expenses are paid, such as rent, payroll and taxes).

Selling Price is the amount the product is sold for once the markup is added to the cost of the product. In the example given the selling price would be $6.00.

Purchase Price is the amount the product cost. In the example given, the cost of the merchandise would be $5.00.

Markup gives the percent that the product is marked up above cost.

Percent markup = $\frac{\textbf{Markup}}{\textbf{Selling Price}}$ **x 100%**

$\frac{\$1.00}{\$6.00}$ x 100% = 17% (Percent markup)

Or

Percent markup = $\frac{\textbf{Selling price - Purchase price}}{\textbf{Selling price}}$ **x 100%**

$\frac{\$6.00 - \$5.00}{\$6.00}$ x 100% = 17% (Percent markup)

Understand the formula:
- **Purchase price** is the AWP (Average Wholesale Price) → the lower number (the cost of merchandise).
- **Selling price** is what the product retails for → the larger number (how much the product is sold for).

Example:

What is the percent markup if Drug A is bought for $10.00 and sold for $17.00?

(% markup) $X = \dfrac{\$17.00 - \$10.00}{\$17.00}$

$X = \dfrac{\$7.00}{\$17.00}$

$X = 0.41$

$0.41 \times 100\% = 41\%$

Practice Problems

1. The AWP for a generic Zoloft 100 mg is $40.12 per bottle of 50 tablets. If the pharmacy retails the product for $55.99, what is the percent markup for this drug?
Markup = Selling Price – Purchase Price
Markup = $55.99 - $40.12 = $15.87
Markup = $15.87

Percent Markup = $\dfrac{\text{Markup}}{\text{Selling price}} \times 100\%$

Percent Markup = $\dfrac{\$15.87}{\$55.99} \times 100\% = 28.3\%$

Percent Markup = 28.3%

2. If the AWP for a drug is $60.00 and the drug retails for $85.00, what is the percent markup for this drug?
Percent Markup = $\dfrac{\text{Markup}}{\text{Selling price}} \times 100\%$

Markup = $85.00 - $60.00 = $25.00

Percent Markup = $\dfrac{\$25.00}{\$85.00} \times 100\% = 29.4\%$

3. If a drug product is acquired for $50.00 and sold for $65.00, what is the percent markup?
Mark up = $65.00 - $50.00 = $15.00

Percent Markup = $\dfrac{\$15.00}{\$65.00} \times 100\% = 23\%$

4. If the AWP for a drug is $67.90 and the drug retails for $85.99, what is the percent markup for this drug?
Markup = $85.99 - $67.90 = $18.09

Percent Markup = $\dfrac{\$18.09}{\$85.99} \times 100\% = 21\%$

Gross Profit:

Gross profit = total sales – purchase price

Example:

If sales were $20,120 for the day and the cost of goods sold were $17,500, what would be the gross profit?

$20,120.00 - $17,500.00 = $2,620.00

Net Profit:

- Gross profit is the difference between the cost of goods sold and how much the merchandise actually cost. The difference between the gross profit and the cost of goods sold is $2,620.00, but this is not the actual or real profit. Net profit takes all overhead into account such as cost of goods sold, payroll, electricity, mortgage etc... So, if gross profit was $2,620.00 and overhead was $830.00, what would be the net profit?
$2,620.00 - $830.00 = $1,790.00
$1,790.00 is the actual, real, or net profit.

CHAPTER 7

TOP

200

DRUGS

TOP 200 DRUGS

Brand	Generic	Indication	Action / Class
Toprol XL	metoprolol succinate	HTN, angina, symptomatic CHF	Selective β1-Blocker
Xanax	alprazolam	Anxiety, panic disorder	Benzodiazepine
Proventil, Ventolin	albuterol	Bronchospasm	β-2 Agonist
Zoloft	sertraline	Depression, OCD, panic disorder, PTSD	SSRI
Zocor	simvastatin	Hyperlipidemia	Statin
Norvasc	amlodipine	HTN	CCB
Glucophage, Glucophage ER	metformin, metformin ER	Type 2 DM	Biguanide antidiabetic
Motrin	ibuprofen	Primary dysmenorrhea, osteoarthritis, rheumatoid arthritis, juvenile arthritis	NSAID
Maxzide, Dyazide	triamterene/hctz	HTN, edema	Diuretic combination
Ambien	zolpidem	Insomnia	GABA-A Receptor Modulator
Keflex	cephalexin	Infection	Cephalosporin
Nexium	esomeprazole	GI ulcer, GERD	PPI
Prevacid	lansoprazole	GI ulcer, GERD	PPI
Lexapro	escitalopram	Depression, GAD	SSRI
Deltasone	prednisone	Allergic & inflammatory diseases, MS acute exacerbations	Steroid
Zyrtec	cetirizine	Allergic rhinitis, chronic idiopathic urticaria	H1-Receptor Antagonist
Singulair	montelukast	Asthma	Leukotriene Receptor Antagonist
Celebrex	celecoxib	Osteoarthritis, rheumatoid arthritis, dysmenhorrhea	COX-2 specific NSAID
Prozac	fluoxetine	Depression, OCD, bulimia nervosa	SSRI
Fosamax	alendronate	Osteoporosis	Bisphosphonate
Lopressor	metoprolol tartrate	HTN, Acute MI	β1-blocker
Levoxyl	levothyroxine	Hypothyroidism	T4 thyroid hormone
Ativan	lorazepam	Anxiety	Benzodiazepine

Protonix	pantoprazole	GI ulcer, GERD	PPI
Elavil	amitriptyline	Depression	TCA
Premarin	conjugated estrogens	menopausal symptoms, female hypogonadism & castration, primary ovarian failure, inoperable breast & prostatic cancer	Estrogens
Allegra	fexofenadine	Allergic rhinitis, chronic idiopathic urticaria	H1-Receptor Antagonist
Plavix	clopidogrel	Reduction of atherosclerotic events	ADP-Inhibitor
Effexor XR, Effexor	venlafaxine ER, venlafaxine	Depression, General Anxiety Disorder	5HT&NE RI, weak DA RI
K-Dur, Klor-Con, Slow K	potassium chloride	Potassium Replacement	Potassium
Darvocet N	propoxyphene/ apap	Narcotic analgesic (CIV)	Weak μ-Opiate Receptor Agonist/ CNS COX-1&2-Inhibitor
Advair	salmeterol/ fluticasone	Asthma, COPD	Long acting β-2 Agonist & Anti-inflammtory Corticosteroid
Coumadin	warfarin	Anticoagulation	Vitamin K-Dependent Factors (II, VII, IX, X) & Protein C,S Synthesis Inhibitor
Tylenol #3	apap w/ codeine	Narcotic analgesic (CIII)	CNS COX-1&2-Inhibitor/ Weak μ-Opiate Receptor Agonist
Klonopin	clonazepam	Lennox-Gastaut syndrome, akinetic & myoclonic seizures, absence seizures	Benzodiazepine
Neurontin	gabapentin	Partial seizure	GABA Analog, MOA unknown
Flonase	fluticasone	Seasonal Allergic Rhinitis	Anti-inflammatory Corticosteroid
Augmentin, Augmentin ES	amoxicillin/ clavulanate, amoxicillin/ clavulanate ES	Infection	Penicillin
Zantac	ranitidine	GI ulcer, GERD	H2-Antagonist

Vasotec	enalapril	HTN, CHF, asymptomatic LVF	ACE-Inhibitor
Paxil, Paxil CR	paroxetine, paroxetine CR	Depression, OCD, panic disorder, SAD	SSRI
Pravachol	pravastatin	Hyperlipidemia, reduce risk of MI	Statin
Viagra	sildenafil	Erectile Dysfunction	PDE5 Inhibitor
Flexeril	cyclobenzaprine	Muscle relaxant	Central action at the brain stem, reduction of tonic somatic motor activity influencing α&γ motorneurons
Altace	ramipril	HTN, reduce risk of MI, CHF	ACE-Inhibitor
Diovan	valsartan	HTN	ARB
Lotrel	amlodipine/ benazepril	HTN	CCB/ACE-Inhibitor combination
Percocet	oxycodone/apap	Narcotic analgesic (CII)	μ-Opiate Receptor Agonist/ CNS COX-1&2-Inhibitor
Valium	diazepam	Anxiety, convulsive disorders, acute alcoholism	Benzodiazepine
Ultram	tramadol	Analgesic	μ opioid-Receptor Agonist, 5HT&NE RI
Calan, Isoptin, Isoptin SR, Verelan	verapamil	HTN, angina	CCB
Diovan HCT	valsartan/hctz	HTN	ARB/Thiazide
Zestoretic	lisinopril/hctz	HTN	ACEI/Thiazide
Ortho-Evra	norelgestromin/ ethinyl estradiol transdermal	Transdermal contraceptive	Inhibit ovulation
Celexa	citalopram	Depression	SSRI
Accupril	quinapril	HTN, Heart Failure	ACE-Inhibitor
Soma	carisoprodol	Muscle relaxant	Central action in the spinal cord
Actos	pioglitazone	Type 2 DM	Thiazolidinediones
Phenergan	promethazine	Nausea/vomitting, sedation, rhinitis, urticaria, motion sickness	H1-Receptor Antagonist
Actonel	risedronate	Osteoporosis	Bisphosphonate
Cozaar	losartan	HTN	ARB
Imdur	isosorbide mononitrate	Angina	Nitrate

Zyloprim	allopurinol	Gout, uric acid nephropathy, secondary hyperuricemia, recurrent calcium oxalate stones	Xanthine oxidase Inhibitor
Catapres	clonidine	HTN	α-2 Receptor Agonist
Cipro	ciprofloxacin	Infection	FQ
Wellbutrin, Wellbutrin XL, Wellbutrin SR	bupropion, bupropion XL, bupropion SR	Depression	DA Reuptake Inhibitor
Micronase, DiaBeta	glyburide	Type 2 DM	Sulfonylurea
Avandia	rosiglitazone	Type 2 DM	Thiazolidinediones
Veetids	penicillin v potassium	Infection	Penicillin
Zetia	ezetimibe	Hyperlipidemia	Inhibits intestinal absorption of cholesterol
Medrol	methyl-prednisolone	Allergic & inflammatory diseases, MS acute exacerbations	Steroid
Folic acid	folacin, pteroylglutamine acid, folate	megaloblastic anemia due to folic acid deficiency, anemias during pregnancy & lactation	Vitamin supplement
Aciphex	rabeprazole	GI ulcer, GERD	PPI
Glucotrol, Glucotrol XL	glipizide, glipzide ER	Type 2 DM	Sulfonylurea
Flomax	tamsulosin	BPH	Selective α-Receptor Blocker
Cardizem, Tiazac, Cardia XT	diltiazem	HTN, angina	CCB
Risperdal	risperidone	Psychotic disorders	5HT2 & DA-Receptors Antagonist
Prilosec	omeprazole	GI ulcer, GERD	PPI
Yasmin	drospirenone/ ethinyl estradiol	OCP	Inhibit ovulation through suppression of LH & FSH
Vibramycin Hyclate	doxycycline hyclate	Infection	Tetracycline
Tricor	fenofibrate	Hyperlipidemia	PPARa agonist
Seroquel	quetiapine	Psychotic disorders	5HT2 & DA-Receptor Antagonist
Lantus	insulin glargine	DM	Insulin

Adderall XR	amphetamine combo	ADHA, narcolepsy	CNS stimulant through release of NE by binding to adrenergic receptors
Concerta	methylphenidate ER	ADHD	CNS stimulant through NE&DA RI
Nasonex	mometasone	Seasonal & Perennial Allergic Rhinitis	Corticosteroid
Clarinex	desloratidine	Nasal and non-nasal symptoms of seasonal, perennial allergic rhinitis; chronic idiopathic urticaria	H1-Receptor Antagonist
Mevacor	lovastatin	Hyperlipidemia	Statin
Hyzaar	losartan/hctz	HTN	ARB/Thiazide combination
Aldactone	spironolactone	essential HTN, edema, hypokalemia, primary hyper aldosteronism	Potassium Sparing Diuretic; aldosterone receptor blocker
Amaryl	glimeperide	Type 2 DM	Sulfonylurea
Lanoxin	digitek, digoxin	CHF, arrythmias	Digitalis glycosides, inhibit Na+/K+ ATPase
Restoril	temazepam	Insomnia	Benzodiazepine
Diflucan	fluconazole	Infection	Sterol inhibitor
Evista	raloxifene	Prevention & treatment of osteoporosis	SERM
Xalatan	latanoprost	Glaucoma	PG Agonist
Coreg	carvedilol	HTN, CHF	Nonselective β & α1-Receptor Blocker
Combivent	albuterol/ ipratropium	COPD	β-2 agonist/ Anticholinergic combination
Crestor	rosuvastatin	Hyperlipidemia	Statin
Valtrex	valacyclovir	genital herpes, Herpes zoster, Varicella zoster	Antiviral
Zyprexa	olanzapine	Psychotic disorders	5HT2 & DA-Receptor Antagonist
Flovent	fluticasone	Asthma	Corticosteroid
Minocin	minocycline	Infection	Tetracycline
Humulin N	insulin NPH	Type 1 & Type 2 DM	Insulin
Prinivil, Zestril	lisinopril	HTN	ACE-Inhibitor
Cardura	doxazosin	BPH, HTN	Selective α1-Receptor Blocker

Oxycontin	oxycodone CR	Narcotic analgesic (CII)	μ-Opiate Receptor Agonist
Kenalog	triamcinolone acetonide	Inflammatory and pruritic dermatoses, inflammatory & ulcerative lesions	Topic Corticosteroid
Estrace	estradiol	menopausal symptoms, female hypogonadism & castration, primary ovarian failure, inoperable breast & prostatic cancer, prevention of menopausal osteoporosis	Estrogen
Allegra-D	fexofenadine w/ pseudoephedrine	Allergic rhinitis	H1-Receptor Antagonist/ Decongestant
Lopid	gemfibrozil	Hyper-triglyceridemia	Fibric Acid
Ortho Tri-Cyclen, Ortho Tri-Cyclen Lo	norgestimate/ ethinyl estradiol	OCP, acne	Inhibit ovulation through suppression of LH & FSH
Reglan	metoclopramide	Diabetic gastroparesis, GERD, prevention of n/v, radiological examinations	DA-Receptor Antagonist
Atarax	hydroxyzine	Anxiety & tension, pruritis, sedative	H1-Receptor Antagonist
Avapro	irbesartan	HTN	ARB
Topamax	topiramate	Partial seizure, tonic-clonic seizures, migraine prevention	GABA-A receptor activation
Imitrex	sumatriptan	Migraine	5HT-1 Receptor Agonist
Straterra	atomoxetine	ADHD	Selective NE RI
Detrol LA	tolteradine	Overactive bladder	Anticholinergic
Omnicef	cefdinir	Infection	Cephalosporin
Antivert	meclizine	Vertigo, motion sickness	H1-Receptor Antagonist
Trinessa	norgestimate/ ethinyl estradiol	OCP	Inhibit ovulation through suppression of LH & FSH
Ultracet	tramadol/apap	Analgesic	μ opioid-Receptor Agonist, 5HT&NE RI/CNS COX-1&2-Inhibitor
Cleocin	clindamycin	Infection	Inhibit protein synthesis
Lotensin	benazepril	HTN	ACE-Inhibitor

Mycostatin	nystatin	Cutaneous or mucotaneous mycotic infections	Binds to sterols in fungal cell membrane, changes membrane permeability, allows leakage of intracellular components
Ziac	bisoprolol/hctz	HTN	Selective β1-blocker/Thiazide combination
Depakote, Depakote ER	divalproex, valproic acid	Simple, complex absence, complex partial seizures, mania, migraine HA prophylaxis	Antiepileptic/ Antipsychotic
Bactrim, Bactrim DS	sulfamethoxazole/ trimethoprim	Infection	Antibacterial/ Sulfonamide
Nasacort AQ	triamcinolone	Seasonal & Perennial Allergic Rhinitis	Corticosteroid
Remeron	mirtazapine	Depression	Central presynaptic α2-Receptor Antagonist
Rhinocort Aqua	budesonide	Seasonal & Perennial Allergic Rhinitis	Glucocorticoid
Inderal, Inderal LA	propranolol, propranolol LA	HTN (SR), arrhythmias, angina (SR), migraine (SR), MI, pheochromocytoma, hypertropic subaortic stenosis	Nonselective β-blocker
Phenergan w/ Codeine	promethazine w/ codeine	Cough & Upper Respiratory symptoms	H1-Receptor Antagonist/Cough suppressant
Hytrin	terazosin	BPH, HTN	α1- Receptor Blocker
Prempro	conjugated estrogens/ medroxy progesterone	menopausal symptoms, prevention of osteoporosis	Estrogen/Progestin combination
Flagyl	metronidazole	Infection	Antibacterial/ Antiprotozoal
Aricept	donepezil	Dementia	Reversible AChE Inhibitor
Buspar	buspirone	Anxiety	Increases NE metabolism, moderate presynaptic DA agonist, 5HT agonist
Mobic	meloxicam	Osteoarthritis	NSAID
Skelaxin	metaxalone	Muscle relaxant	CNS depressant
Duragesic	fentanyl	Narcotic analgesic (CII)	μ-Opiate Receptor Agonist

Zovirax	acyclovir	Genital herpes, chickenpox, Herpes zoster, Varicella zoster	Antiviral
Pepcid	famotidine	GI ulcer, GERD	H2-Receptor Antagonist
Niaspan	niacin, niacinamide	Hyperlipidemia	Increases lipoprotein lipase
Necon	norethindrone/ ethinyl estradiol	OCP	Inhibit ovulation through suppression of LH & FSH
Aviane	levonorgestrel/ ethinyl estradiol	OCP	Inhibit ovulation through suppression of LH & FSH
Voltaren	diclofenac	osteoarthritis, rheumatoid arthritis, ankylosing spondylitis	NSAID
Humalog	insulin lispro	Type 1 & Type 2 DM	Insulin
Elidel	pimecrolimus	Mild to moderate atopic dermatitis	Binds to FKBP-12, inhibits calcineurin; blocks T cell activation
Patanol	olopatadine	Allergic conjunctivitis	H1-Receptor Antagonist (Ophthalmic agent)
Benicar	olmesartan	HTN	ARB
Lotrisone	clotrimazole/ betamethasone	Tinea cruris, corporis, pedis	Topical antifungal/ Adrenocorticoid
Biaxin XL, Biaxin	clarithromycin XL, clarithromycin	Infection	Macrolide
Tri-Sprintec	norgestimate/ ethinyl estradiol	OCP	Inhibit ovulation through suppression of LH & FSH
Rheumatrex, Trexall	methotrexate	Trophoblastic neoplasms, leukemias, psoriasis, rheumatoid arthritis, carcinomas, osteosarcomas, lymphomas	Inhibits DNA synthesis through binding to DHFR, inhibiting the formation of reduced folates & thymidylate synthesis
Lamictal	lamotrigine	Partial seizures, adjunct in generalized seizures	Stabilization of neuronal membranes, modulation of presynaptic transmitter release of excitatory amino acids
Pamelor	nortriptyline	Depression	TCA
Qualaquin	quinine sulfate	Malaria	Depresses oxygen uptake and carbohydrate

Dilantin	phenytoin	Tonic-clonic, psychomotor seizures	Antiepileptic
Monopril	fosinopril	HTN, CHF	ACE-Inhibitor
Miralax, Glycolax	polyethylene glycol	Constipation	Induces catharsis by strong electrolyte and osmotic effects
Pulmicort	budesonide	Asthma	Anti-inflammatory Corticosteroid
Nizoral	ketoconazole	Infection	Impairs the synthesis of ergosterol
Avalide	irbesartan/hctz	HTN	ARB/Thiazide combination
Ditropan XL	oxybutinin XL	Overactive bladder, bladder instability	Anticholinergic
Zyrtec-D	cetirizine w/ pseudoephedrine	Allergic rhinitis, chronic idiopathic urticaria	H1-Receptor Antagonist/ Decongestant
Macrobid	nitrofurantoin monohydrate	Infection	Inhibitor of Acetyl CoA & metabolism of bacterial carbohydrates
Zanaflex	tizanidine	Muscle relaxant	α2-Agonist, increases presynaptic inhibition of motor neurons
Provera	medroxy progesterone	Abnormal uterine bleeding, secondary amenorrhea, reduction of endometrial hyperplasia	Progestin hormone
Glucovance	metformin/ glyburide	Type 2 DM	Biguanide antidiabetic/ Sulfonylurea
Timoptic	timolol	Glaucoma	Nonselective β-blocker; reduces aqueous humor formation and increases outflow
Capoten	captopril	HTN, CHF, nephropathy, prevention of kidney failure, increase survival rate post MI	ACE-Inhibitor
Adalat CC	nifedipine ER	HTN	CCB
Sinemet	carbidopa/ levodopa	Parkinson's	Levodopa decarboxylation Inhibitor/Precursor of DA
Humulin 70/30	NPH insulin/ Regular insulin	Type 1 & Type 2 DM	Insulin

Microgestin FE	norethindrone/ ethinyl estradiol	OCP	Inhibit ovulation through suppression of LH & FSH
Relafen	nabumetone	osteoarthritis, rheumatoid arthritis	NSAID
Anusol	hydrocortisone	Hemorrhoids, chronic UC	Steroid
Luminal	phenobarbital	Seizure, sedation, hypnosis	Antiepileptic, Hypnotic
Levsin	hyoscyamine sulfate	peptic ulcer, IBS, neurogenic bladder/bowel disorders, gastric hyperspasmodic & hypersecretory disorders, rhinitis	Anticholinergic
Pyridium	phenazopyridine	UTI analgesic	unknown MOA
Apri	desogestrel/ ethinyl estradiol	OCP	Inhibit ovulation
Kariva	desogestrel/ ethinyl estradiol	OCP	Inhibit ovulation
Nolvadex	tamoxifen	Metastatic breast cancer in men, postmenopausal women, delaying recurrence following total mastectomy, axillary dissection, reduction incidence in high risk women	Antineoplastic/ Antiestrogen
Avelox	moxifloxacin	Infection	FQ
Lescol XL	fluvastatin XL	Hyperlipidemia	Statin
Proscar	finasteride	BPH	5-α Reductase Inhibitor and decreasing 5-α-DHT conversion from testosterone
Robaxin	methocarbamol	Muscle relaxant	Central action in the spinal cord, inhibiting the flexor & crossed extensor reflexes
Vicodin, Vicodin ES, Vicodin HP, Lortab, Norco, Lorcet, Lorcet Plus	hydrocodone/apap	Narcotic analgesic (CIII)	
Lipitor	atorvastatin	Hyperlipidemia	Statin
Tenormin	atenolol	HTN, angina, acute MI	Selective β1-Blocker

Synthroid	levothyroxine	Hypothyroidism	T4 thyroid hormone
Amoxil, Trimox	amoxicillin	Infection	Penicillin
HydroDIURIL, Esidrix	hctz	HTN, edema	Thiazide Diuretic
Zithromax	azithromycin	Infection	Macrolide
Lasix	furosemide	HTN, edema	Loop Diuretic
Indocin	indomethacin	osteoarthritis, rheumatoid arthritis, ankylosing spondylitis,	NSAID
Lithonate	lithium carbonate	Psychotic disorders	Antagonism of NE and DA release from nerve terminals, increases reuptake and inactivation of catecholamines
Tessalon	benzonatate	Cough	Antitussive through anesthetizing stretch receptors in the respiratory passages
Tenoretic	atenolol/ chlorthalidone	HTN	Selective β1-blocker/Diuretic combination
Naprosyn	naproxen	pain, dysmenorrhea, acute tendinitis & bursitis, rheumatoid & osteoarthritis, ankylosing spondilits, acute gout	NSAID
Levaquin	levofloxacin	Infection	FQ
Desyrel	trazodone	Depression	5HT-RI

Abbreviations:

Statin = HMG CoA Reductase Inhibitor   ARB = Angiotensin Receptor Blocker

ACE-Inhibitor = Angiotensin Converting Enzyme Inhibitor

SSRI = Selective Serotonin Reuptake Inhibitor   PPI = Proton Pump Inhibitor

CCB = Calcium Channel Blocker   FQ = Fluoroquinolone

TCA = Tricyclic Antidepressant   DHFR = Dihydrofolate Reductase

NSAID = Nonsteroidal Anti-inflammatory Drug

PABA = Para-aminobenzoic acid   PDE5- Inhibitor = Phosphodiesterase 5 Inhibitor
AChE Inhibitor = Acetylcholinesterase Inhibitor

H1-Receptor Antagonist = Histamine 1 Receptor Antagonist

ADP Inhibitor = Adenosine Diphosphate Inhibitor

5HT&NE&DA RI = Serotonin & Norephinephrine & Dopamine Reuptake Inhibitor

H2-Receptor Antagonist = Histamine 2 Receptor Antagonist

PPARa Agonist = Peroxisome Proliferator Activated Receptor a Agonist

5HT RI = Serotonin Reuptake Inhibitor   SERM = Selective Estrogen Receptor Modulator

PRACTICE

TESTS

CHAPTER 8

PRACTICE TESTS

Practice Test #1

1. Flecanide 100 mg, po tablet, bid #60. Which statement is false?
   - a. The directions state to take one tablet by mouth twice daily
   - b. Tambocor is the brand name for Flecanide
   - c. Flecanide is an antiarrythmic
   - d. Flecanide only comes in a patch dosage form

2. What drug would be used for convulsive disorders?
   - a. Depakote
   - b. Coreg
   - c. Imitrex
   - d. Digoxin

3. Actonel and Fosamax are used for which disease state?
   - a. Osteoporosis
   - b. Arthritis
   - c. Rhinitis
   - d. Overactive bladder

4. Topamax 25 mg, 1 po qd. Which statement is false?
   - a. The directions state to instill one drop into each eye
   - b. Topamax is used for epilepsy and migraine headaches
   - c. The generic name for Topamax is Topiramate
   - d. Topamax 25 mg comes in a capsule and tablet dosage form

5. How many 500 mg doses would be contained in 10 gm of amoxicillin?
   - a. 5
   - b. 10
   - c. 15
   - d. 20

6. Which of the following drugs is exempt from the Poision Prevention Act?
   - a. Viagra
   - b. Levsin sublingual tablets
   - c. Nitrogloycerin sublingual tablets
   - d. Tussionex suspension

7. A patient using Vancomycin should be monitored for _____.
   - a. Nephrotoxicity
   - b. Ototoxicity
   - c. Both a and b
   - d. None of the above

8. Which counseling tip should be given to a patient taking Flagyl (Metronidazole)?
   - a. Avoid alcohol while taking this medication
   - b. Must take with vitamin B6
   - c. Do not take with NSAID's
   - d. All of the above

9. Rx   Carbamide Peroxide   6.5%
   Glycerin   ad   60 mL
   Sig. Five drops in right ear.
   How many grams of carbamide peroxide should be used to prepare this prescription?
   - a. 3.9 gm
   - b. 2.3 gm
   - c. 7 gm
   - d. 11 gm

10. Fluconazole i po stat. Which statement is true?
    a. Fluconazole is an antifungal
    b. Fluconazole is an antibiotic
    c. Fluconazole is an antihelmith
    d. Fluconazole is an antiviral

11. PCN 500 mg i po stat, then i po q6h ug. Which statement is false?
    a. Penicillin is in the same family as Augmentin
    b. Penicillin is in the same family as Amoxicillin
    c. Penicillin is in the same family as Biaxin
    d. The directions state to take one tablet now, and then take 1 tablet every 6 hours until all taken

12. When dispensing NSAID's, birth control and accutane, how often should a med guide be included?
    a. Just with the original prescription
    b. Only if the patient requests one
    c. Every time the prescription is filled or refilled
    d. Never, they are generally safe drugs

13. Which agency regulates medical devices?
    a. DEA
    b. EPA
    c. DPS
    d. FDA

14. Which drug is not a controlled drug substance?
    a. Acebutolol
    b. Oxycontin
    c. Lorazepam
    d. Daytrana

15. Which drug has a major side effect of constipation?
    a. Iron
    b. Verapamil
    c. Morphine
    d. All of the above

16. Which one of the following drugs does not cause photosensitivity?
    a. Cipro
    b. Septra
    c. Levofloxacin
    d. Amoxicillin

17. Which drug is not a benzodiazepine?
    a. Lorazepam
    b. Valium
    c. Ultram
    d. Clonazepam

18. Accupril is in which drug classification?
    a. Beta blocker
    b. ACE inhibitor
    c. Calcium channel blocker
    d. Angiotensin II receptor antagonist

19. Rx   Keralac®   50%
    Compound Benzoin Tincture ad 50 mL
    Sig. Apply to area of dry skin TID.
    How many grams of Keralac® should be used to prepare this prescription?
    a. 0.25 gm
    b. 25 gm
    c. 12.5 gm
    d. 250 gm

20. Nasonex, Miacalcin and Flonase are administered by which route of administration?
  a. Oral
  b. Rectal
  c. Nasal
  d. In the ear

21. If a patient cannot take an NSAID due to a previous allergic reaction, they should be counseled to take which of the following drugs for mild pain?
  a. Acetaminophen
  b. Naproxen
  c. Meloxicam
  d. Ketoprofen

22. If a patient is allergic to opioids, they should not take which of the following drugs?
  a. Ultram
  b. Depakote
  c. Morphine
  d. Lisinopril

23. Morphine is in which controlled drug substance schedule?
  a. CI
  b. CII
  c. CIII
  d. CIV

24. Cocaine is in which controlled drug substance schedule?
  a. CI
  b. CII
  c. CIII
  d. CIV

25. Morphine is a/an _____.
  a. Stimulant
  b. Narcotic
  c. Benzodiazepine
  d. Barbiturate

26. Which drug should be kept in its original container?
  a. Nitroglycerin sublingual tablets
  b. Seizure medications
  c. Control substances
  d. All of the above

27. What is the maximum amount of Acetaminophen that should be consumed daily?
  a. 1000 mg
  b. 2000 mg
  c. 3000 mg
  d. 4000 mg

28. When the word "sig" is seen on a prescription, what does it mean?
  a. The directions for the patient
  b. To check the patient's allergies
  c. Patient's address
  d. Doctor's address

29. How many ml of 90% Dextrose should be mixed with water to make 1 liter of a 30% Dextrose solution?
  a. 118 ml of 90% Dextrose
  b. 237 ml of 90% Dextrose
  c. 333 ml of 90% Dextrose
  d. 476 ml of 90% Dextrose

30. Phenergan 25 mg, 1 po q 4-6 h prn n/v. Which statement is false?
   a. The directions state to take one tablet by mouth every 4 to 6 hours as needed for nausea and vomiting
   b. The generic name for Phenergan is Promethazine
   c. The directions state insert one suppository rectally every 4 to 6 hours as needed for nausea and vomiting
   d. Phenergan is used for nausea and vomiting

31. The term "before meals" would use which Latin abbreviation?
   a. ou
   b. pc
   c. ac
   d. qd

32. What does the abbreviation "APAP" refer to?
   a. Allergy
   b. Acetaminophen
   c. After meals
   d. Antihistamine

33. On a prescription that reads "Promethazine 25 mg pr q6h prn n/v", which dosage form would be dispensed?
   a. Suppositories
   b. Drops
   c. Tablets
   d. Elixer

34. What filter size would be considered a sterilizing filter?
   a. 0.11 micron
   b. 0.22 micron
   c. 0.31 micron
   d. 0.42 micron

35. Which type of drug would be placed under the tongue?
   a. Enteric coated
   b. Buccal
   c. Sublingual
   d. Delayed release

36. Where would a buccal tablet be placed?
   a. Rectally
   b. Under the tongue
   c. Swallowed and dissolved in the intestine
   d. Inside the cheek

37. Robaxin 750 mg, 1 po tid prn for muscle cramps. Which statement is false?
   a. The generic for Robaxin is Metformin
   b. The directions state to take one tablet by mouth 3 times daily as needed for muscle cramps
   c. Robaxin is a muscle relaxant
   d. Robaxin comes in tablet and injection dosage forms

38. The highest concentration of alcohol would be contained in which type of formulation?
   a. Solution
   b. Suspension
   c. Syrup
   d. Tincture

39. If an injection contains 1% (w/v) of diphenhydramine, calculate the number of milligrams of the drug in 50 mL of injection.
    a. 100 mg
    b. 250 mg
    c. 1000 mg
    d. 500 mg
40. Which of the following drugs would be listed on a DEA 222 form?
    a. Xanax
    b. Soma
    c. Ritalin
    d. Vicodin
41. Which drug comes in a patch and a tablet dosage form?
    a. Clonidine
    b. Topamax
    c. Accupril
    d. Benadryl
42. How many milligrams of Zantac 15 mg/ml would be contained in 350 ml?
    a. 3640 mg
    b. 5250 mg
    c. 23 mg
    d. 230 mg
43. Which of the following eye drops must be refrigerated?
    a. Tobrex
    b. Floxin
    c. Ocuflox
    d. Xalatan
44. Which drug would be the safest choice to reduce fever in a patient with peptic ulcer disease?
    a. Acteaminophen
    b. Ibuprofen
    c. Naproxen
    d. Aspirin
45. Which of the following drugs is an antihistamine that can be used to treat itching?
    a. Hydroxyzine
    b. Diphenhydramine
    c. Loratidine
    d. All of the above
46. What would be the best way to dispose of used needles?
    a. Regular trash
    b. Wrap needle up in a plastic bag
    c. Place needle in a sharp's container
    d. Break off needle and place in regular trash
47. Omnicef 300 mg, 1 po bid ug. Which statement is false?
    a. Omnicef is an antibiotic
    b. The directions state to take one by mouth twice daily until all taken
    c. Cefdinir is the generic name for Omnicef
    d. Omnicef is a Penicillin antibiotic
48. A prescription drug is also known as which of the following?
    a. Legend drug
    b. OTC drug
    c. Orphan drug
    d. All of the above
49. How many ml of 70% ethanol should be mixed with water to make 1 liter of 50% ethanol solution?
    a. 714 ml 70%
    b. 209 ml 70%
    c. 650 ml 70%
    d. 625 ml 70%

50. Which of the following is not part of a syringe?
    a. Barrel
    b. Luer-lock tip
    c. Plunger
    d. All of the above are parts of a syringe
51. If a patient is using 33 units of NPH what size syringe should be used?
    a. 0.3 cc
    b. 0.5 cc
    c. 1.0 cc
    d. None of the above
52. If a patient taking coumadin has a high fever, which medication should they be counseled to take?
    a. Acetaminophen
    b. Ibuprofen
    c. Naproxen
    d. Aspirin
53. Benzodiazepines are in which controlled drug substance schedule?
    a. CI
    b. CII
    c. CIII
    d. CIV
54. Which of the following is incorrect when counseling patients who are taking HMG-CoA reductase inhibitors ("statins")?
    a. Do not become pregnant while taking this medication
    b. May cause rhabdomyolysis
    c. Usually taken at night
    d. It is not important to monitor LFT's (liver function test)
55. Niacin is which B vitamin?
    a. B1
    b. B2
    c. B3
    d. B12
56. How many gallons are contained in 120 pints?
    a. 5 gallons
    b. 15 gallons
    c. 7.5 gallons
    d. 23 gallons
57. Acyclovir is classified as which type of drug?
    a. Antibiotic
    b. Antiviral
    c. Antineoplastic
    d. Hyperlipidemic
58. Which statement is not true regarding fluoroquinolones?
    a. Should not be given to children due to bone formation problems
    b. Are considered narrow spectrum antibiotics
    c. Should not be taken with iron, antacids or vitamins
    d. May cause photosensitivity
59. Which drug is not considered a macrolide antibiotic?
    a. Clarithromycin
    b. Clindamycin
    c. Azithromycin
    d. Erythromycin
60. Which drug class will have a cross sensitivity type reaction with penicillin?
    a. Macrolides
    b. Fluoroquinolones
    c. Aminoglycosides
    d. Cephalosporins

61. Medrol dose pack, uad. Which statement is false?
    a. The directions state to take as directed
    b. Methylprednisolone is the generic name for Medrol
    c. Medrol is an antibiotic
    d. Medrol dose pack is usually given as a tapering dose regimen
62. Lasix 40 mg 1 po bid. Which statement about Lasix is false?
    a. The generic name of Lasix is Bumetanide
    b. The generic name of Lasix is Furosemide
    c. The directions state to take one tablet by mouth twice daily
    d. Lasix is a loop diurectic
63. Which drug is considered a narcotic?
    a. Dextromethorphan
    b. Lorazepam
    c. Benzonatate
    d. Codeine
64. The physician orders 250 ml of heparin to be infused over 15 hours. How many ml/hr should the IV pump be programmed for?
    a. 3.5 ml/hr
    b. 22.3 ml/hr
    c. 12.25 ml/hr
    d. 16.7 ml/hr
65. Which insulin comes in an inhalation dosage form?
    a. Humulin R (insulin regular)
    b. Exubera (insulin human)
    c. Humulin N (insulin isophane NPH)
    d. Byetta (Exenatide)
66. Subcutaneously (SC) refers to which type of injection?
    a. Directly under the skin
    b. Deep muscle injection
    c. Into the vein
    d. Into the heart
67. The correct statement concerning drug recalls is:
    a. There are 3 classifications of drug recalls 1 being the least serious and 3 being the most serious.
    b. There are 4 classifications of drug recalls 1 being the most serious and 4 being the least serious.
    c. There are 3 classifications of drug recalls 1 being the most serious and 3 being the least serious.
    d. There are 5 classifications of drug recalls 1 being the least serious and 5 being the most serious.
68. What is the medication list that a practitioner may prescribe from in a hospital setting called?
    a. Formulary
    b. Drug listing
    c. DEA 106 list
    d. JACHO drug listing
69. It is legal for an optometrist to prescribe drugs for an upper respirtory tract infection.
    a. True
    b. False
70. Levaquin 750 mg, 1 po qd. Which statement is false?
    a. The directions state to take one tablet by mouth every day
    b. Levaquin is a broad spectrum antibiotic
    c. Levaquin can cause photosensitivity and should not be taken with iron, antacids and vitamins
    d. The generic name for Levaquin is Ciprofloxacin

71. What is 20% of 200?
    a. 10
    b. 20
    c. 30
    d. 40

72. USPDI volume I contains:
    a. Drug information written for the health care provider
    b. Drug information written for patients
    c. Therapeutic equivalency information
    d. Pharmacy law

73. A drug monograph gives information on which of the following?
    a. Chemical structures
    b. Drug information
    c. Drugs that are soon to be released
    d. A drug's cost and AWP

74. Controlled drug substances schedule I drugs:
    a. Are rarely dispensed due to their highly addictive properties
    b. Are the least addictive of all the control substances
    c. Require a special prescription from a doctor
    d. Have no accepted medicinal use

75. Combat Methamphetamine Epidemic Act (CMEA):
    a. Limits the purchase of pseudoephedrine.
    b. Allows the patient to purchase 3.6 gm of pseudoephedrine per day
    c. Allows the patient to purchase 9 gm of pseudoephedrine per 30 days
    d. All of the above

76. A patient may receive a refill for which of the following drugs?
    a. Valium
    b. Oxycontin
    c. Ritalin
    d. Concerta

77. The discontinuation of Bextra would be classified as a _____.
    a. Voluntary discontinuation
    b. Class I recall
    c. Class II recall
    d. Class III recall

78. One of the purposes of a state board of pharmacy is to protect which of the following?
    a. The doctor
    b. The pharmacist
    c. The public
    d. All of the above

79. Which size beaker should be used when measuring 8 ml of liquid?
    a. 3 ml
    b. 5 ml
    c. 10 ml
    d. 20 ml

80. In what proportion should 30% zinc oxide ointment be mixed with an ointment base to produce a 5% zinc oxide ointment?
    a. 1:5
    b. 1:10
    c. 1:50
    d. 1:100

81. A patient that has received and overdose of warfarin should receive which vitamin to increase blood clotting factors?
   a. Vitamin B
   b. Vitamin C
   c. Vitamin K
   d. Vitamin A

82. What federal agency would lost or stolen control drug substances be reported to?
   a. DEA
   b. DPS
   c. OSHA
   d. JACHO

83. Who would have the authorization to change the drug formulary?
   a. Pharmacy and Therapeutics Committee (P&T Committee)
   b. Administration counsel
   c. Board of directors
   d. None of the above

84. Which drug recall goes to the customer level (pharmacist contacts customer)?
   a. Recall I
   b. Recall II
   c. Recall III
   d. All recalls go to the customer level

85. Which drug would not be considered a controlled drug substance schedule CI?
   a. LSD
   b. Cocaine
   c. Peyote
   d. Marijuana

86. Which DEA form is proof of receipt of controlled drug substance schedule CII's?
   a. DEA 41
   b. DEA 106
   c. DEA 222
   d. DEA 224

87. Which drug does not require refrigeration?
   a. Xalatan
   b. Insulin
   c. Miacalcin
   d. Tobrex

88. How any milliliters of 70% alcohol should be mixed with a 10% alcohol solution to make 4500 ml of a 30% alcohol solution?
   a. 500 ml
   b. 1000 ml
   c. 1500 ml
   d. 2500 ml

89. Which doctor DEA number is correct?
   a. AS5485481
   b. BS6322684
   c. AB8236547
   d. BS2546987

90. Which doctor DEA number is correct?
   a. BJ1564987
   b. AJ2154872
   c. BJ3889156
   d. AJ2145877

91. Which of the following drugs is a generic name?
    a. Keflex
    b. Voltaren
    c. Cefprozil
    d. Dilantin
92. Milk or diary products should not be taken with which of the following antibiotics?
    a. Amoxicillin
    b. Tetracycline
    c. Cefaclor
    d. Bactrim
93. A pharmacy technician may perform which of the following duties?
    a. Counsel patients on drug-to-drug interactions
    b. Receive and input a CII prescription
    c. Advise a patient on what drug would be best used for a ring worm infection
    d. Counsel a patient on what drugs can be used during pregnancy
94. When using a 150 mg/ml solution, what volume would be needed to give a dose of 0.0750 gm?
    a. 0.5 ml
    b. 1 ml
    c. 0.25 ml
    d. 2 ml
95. Which of the following drugs is a COX-2 inhibitor that is used to treat osteoarthritis?
    a. Zolpidem
    b. Megestrol Acetate
    c. Celecoxib
    d. Lindane
96. Label instructions for Furosemide call for the addition of 9 mL of water to make 10 mL of reconstituted liquid such that each 5 mL contains 100 mg of Furosemide. How much volume is occupied by the dry powder?
    a. 1 ml
    b. 5 ml
    c. 14 ml
    d. 100 ml
97. From the previous question, what is the total amount of Furosemide in the 10 mL product?
    a. 2 mg
    b. 200 mg
    c. 100 mg
    d. 5 mg
98. Using the answer from the previous question, if a doctor orders a furosemide concentration of 75 mg/5 mL (rather than 100 mg/5 mL), how many milliliters of water should be added to the dry powder?
    a. 2 ml
    b. 5 ml
    c. 7.4 ml
    d. 12.33 ml
99. Loperamide is a/an _____.
    a. Laxative
    b. Antitussive
    c. Antidiarrheal agent
    d. Antihistamine
100. How much would 54 tablets of Ferrous Sulfate 325mg cost if a 1000 tablets cost $15.30?
    a. $1.16
    b. $2.54
    c. $8.36
    d. $0.83

101. Ferrous Sulfate 325 mg is equivalent to how many grains:
   a. 2 grains
   b. 5 grains
   c. 7 grains
   d. 10 grains

102. How is Byetta stored?
   a. In the refrigerator
   b. Locked up with the CII drugs
   c. With the liquids
   d. At room temperature

103. Grinding a substance into a very fine powder is a process called _____.
   a. levigation
   b. trituration
   c. emulsion
   d. effervescent

104. Vicodin is in which controlled drug substance schedule?
   a. Schedule I
   b. Schedule II
   c. Schedule III
   d. Schedule IV

105. Oxycontin is in which controlled drug substance schedule?
   a. Schedule I
   b. Schedule II
   c. Schedule III
   d. Schedule IV

106. Heroin is in which controlled drug substance schedule?
   a. Schedule I
   b. Schedule II
   c. Schedule III
   d. Schedule IV

107. Turnover rate refers to:
   a. The amount of inventory being replaced in a specific amount of time
   b. How quickly medication is going out-of-date
   c. On average how much time it will take medication to go out-of-date
   d. None of the above

108. Which document would be used as proof of receipt of a CIII controlled substance?
   a. Blue copy of a 222 form
   b. Green copy of a 222 form
   c. Commercial invoice
   d. Control inventory report

109. In a situation where state and federal law conflict, which law should take precedence?
   a. Shortest time period for record retention
   b. Longest time period for record retention
   c. Follow state law
   d. Follow federal law

110. A patient that is allergic to both Amoxicillin and Cephalexin would be said to have what type of reaction?
   a. Allergic reaction
   b. This is the side effects of the medications
   c. Hypersensitivity reaction
   d. Cross-sensitivity reaction

111. What is the filter size of a filter needle?
   a. 5 micron
   b. 2 micron
   c. 1 micron
   d. 7 micron

112. Which of the following is not true regarding a doctors DEA number?
    a. Needed on all prescriptions
    b. Is coded to prevent forgery
    c. Is needed for controlled substances
    d. Is specific for each doctor
113. To what governmental agency should adverse drug reactions and outcomes be reported to?
    a. DEA
    b. FDA
    c. DPS
    d. AMA
114. Maintaining patient's profiles is extremely important and is usually done by _____.
    a. Secondary agency
    b. Insurance agencies
    c. Filing system
    d. Daily back-up tape
115. Restoril is used for _____.
    a. Leg cramps
    b. Itching
    c. Fever
    d. Insomnia
116. Restoril is classified as a _____.
    a. OTC medication
    b. Non-controlled drug substance
    c. Drug that requires a package insert
    d. Controlled drug substance schedule IV
117. A prescription is written for Robitussin-AC, 1 teaspoonful by mouth every 6 hours with a quantity of 240 ml. How many days will this medication last if taken as directed?
    a. 6 days
    b. 10 days
    c. 12 days
    d. 14 days
118. Which of the following are fat soluble vitamins?
    a. A, D, E and K
    b. A, B, E and K
    c. B, C, D and E
    d. A, C, D and E
119. How is a buccal tablet given?
    a. Under the tongue
    b. Rectally
    c. Between the cheek and gum
    d. Vaginally
120. Which of the following is not a B vitamin?
    a. Riboflavin
    b. Niacin
    c. Tocopherol
    d. Cyanocobalamin
121. Which route of administration can nitroglycerin be given?
    a. Sublingual (under the tongue)
    b. Transdermal patch
    c. Orally
    d. All of the above
122. Which of the following two drugs are classified in the same family?
    a. Claritin and Pseudoephedrine
    b. Atenolol and Tramadol
    c. Lovastatin and Zocor
    d. Amoxicillin and Levaquin

123. What is the maximum number of refills that can be given for control drug substance schedules CIII - CV by federal law?
    a. One
    b. Five
    c. Six
    d. One year

124. How often should Fosamax 70 mg be given?
    a. Every 4 hours
    b. Once daily
    c. Once weekly
    d. Once monthly

125. The term PO on a prescription refers to?
    a. How often the medication is to be taken
    b. The route of administration
    c. The time the medication should be taken
    d. The quantity to be dispensed

126. A drug that reduces the viscosity of mucus in the lungs and reduces chest congestion is referred to as?
    a. Expectorant
    b. Antihistamine
    c. Antitussive
    d. Antipyretic

127. Dextromethorphan relieves which symptoms?
    a. Runny nose
    b. Chest congestion
    c. Cough
    d. Headache

128. Antipyretic is a term that refers to which condition?
    a. Headache
    b. Fever
    c. Sore throat
    d. Nausea and Vomiting

129. Which of the following drugs must be purchased using a DEA 222 form?
    a. Methadone
    b. Percodan
    c. Methylin
    d. All of the above

130. A drug given directly into the bloodstream is given by which route of administration?
    a. Subcutaneously
    b. Intravenous
    c. Intramuscularly
    d. None of the above

131. How many numbers are in an NDC number?
    a. 5 to 6
    b. 7 to 8
    c. 9 to 10
    d. 10 to 11

132. How much amoxicillin suspension 200 mg/5 ml is required for a dose of 250 mg?
    a. 5ml
    b. 6.25ml
    c. 10ml
    d. 3.125ml

133. A Prescription is written for Synthroid 50mcg #30, SIG: 1qd. The pharmacy has 0.025 mg tablets in stock. The number of tablets dispensed would be:
    a. 30
    b. 15
    c. 6
    d. 60
134. Which of the following actions should be taken if a technician takes a call from a patient whose child has accidently swallowed a pill found on the floor:
    a. Recommend the child be given a lot of water to flush out the drug
    b. Recommend calling the poison control center
    c. Immediately refer the call to the pharmacist
    d. Recommend the patient go to the emergency room
135. Phenobarbital has a recommended storage temperature of _____.
    a. -20 degrees C to -10 degrees C (-4 degrees F to 14 degrees F)
    b. 15 degrees C to 30 degrees C (59 degrees F to 86 degrees F)
    c. 30 degreees C to 40 degrees C (86 degrees F to 104 degrees F)
    d. 8 degrees C to 15 degrees C (46 degrees F to 59 degrees F)
136. If an insurance company will pay for a 30 day supply and the prescription reads " i-ii q 6-8 h," what is the maximum number of units that can be dispensed?
    a. 240
    b. 120
    c. 30
    d. 360
137. An IV infusion order is received for Vancomycin 1000 mg in 1000 mL of NS, to be infused over 90 minutes. What will the flow rate be in mL/min?
    a. 2.2 ml/min
    b. 5.4 ml/min
    c. 11.11 ml/min
    d. 13.25 ml/min
138. A prescription calls for amoxicillin capsules to be administered 1q 6h. The first dose was taken at 10:00 AM. The patient should take the next two doses at?
    a. 2.00 PM and 7.00 PM
    b. 5.00 PM and 11.00 PM
    c. 4.00 PM and 10.00 PM
    d. 10.00 PM and 4.00 AM
139. Omeprazole is the generic name for:
    a. Demerol
    b. Prilosec
    c. Lopid
    d. Valtrex
140. Which of the following drugs must be stored in the refrigerator?
    a. Tegretol
    b. Desyrel
    c. Zyprexa
    d. Xalatan
141. An administration set that delivers 15 gtt/mL infuses 500 mL D5W over a 12 hour period. What flow rate will be required to deliver the 500 mL?
    a. 10.4 gtt/min
    b. 5.5 gtt/min
    c. 7.8 gtt/min
    d. 10.5 gtt/min
142. How many 500 mg doses are contained in a 100 mL bottle of 250 mg/ 5 mL Amoxicillin suspension?
    a. 3
    b. 6
    c. 10
    d. 7

143. What is the error percentage rate if 15 errors are detected in the preparation of 250 prescriptions?
    a. 2%
    b. 10%
    c. 6%
    d. 25%
144. Which of the following drugs is classified as a Schedule II controlled substance?
    a. Haldol
    b. Soma
    c. Xanax
    d. Daytrana
145. A patient with a sulfa allergy will most likely react to which of the following drugs?
    a. Vicodin
    b. Diflucan
    c. Bactrim
    d. Paxil
146. Which of the following drugs should be protected from light?
    a. Tambacor
    b. Oxaprozin
    c. Lunesta
    d. Macrobid
147. If the recommended dose of a medication is 90 mg/kg/day in two divided doses, what dose would be given to a 40 lb child?
    a. 250 mg bid
    b. 375 mg bid
    c. 875 mg bid
    d. 818 mg bid
148. An otic preparation would be placed in the _____.
    a. Ear
    b. Eyes
    c. Mouth
    d. Nose
149. The last two digits of an NDC number represent which of the following?
    a. Manufacturer
    b. Unit package size
    c. Product strength
    d. Dosage form
150. How many grams would be administered when a drug order calls for 10 ml of a 20% solution?
    a. 200 gm
    b. 2 gm
    c. 0.2 gm
    d. 2 mg

Practice Test #2

1. How are ophthalmic drops administered?
   a. By mouth
   b. In the ear
   c. In the eye
   d. On the toenails or fingernails

2. Sublingual, seroquels and spanules are given by which route of administration?
   a. Rectally
   b. Vaginally
   c. By mouth
   d. Topically

3. Which of the following statements is false concerning Ambien?
   a. The generic for Ambien is Zolpidem.
   b. Ambien is a Controlled Drug Substance schedule CIV.
   c. Ambien is used to help patients fall asleep.
   d. White blood cell counts must be monitored while patient is taking this medication.

4. Who approves changes in a hospital's formulary?
   a. DEA
   b. Pharmacy and therapeutics committee (P & T)
   c. Drug review committee
   d. OSHA

5. What is the generic name for Motrin?
   a. Naproxen
   b. Ketoprofen
   c. Celebrex
   d. Ibuprofen

6. What adverse event may occur if Flagyl (metronidazole) and alcohol are taken together?
   a. Joint pain
   b. Antabuse type reaction
   c. Blurred vision
   d. Weight loss

7. Prednisone 5 mg, day 1 & 2 40 mg qd, day 2 & 3 30mg qd, day 4 & 5 20 mg qd, day 6 & 7 10 mg qd, day 7 & 8 5 mg qd

   How many 5mg tablets must be dispensed?
   a. 50 tablets
   b. 42 tablets
   c. 32 tablets
   d. 28 tablets

8. How often should a HEPA filter be inspected?
   a. Every month
   b. Every 3 months
   c. Every 6 months
   d. Every year

9. Cipro 500 mg, i po bid x 7d. Which statement is false?
   a. Children should never take this drug orally.
   b. "Floxacin" is in the suffix for the generic name of this drug
   c. This drug is a flouroquinolone broad spectrum antibiotic.
   d. The directions state to take one tablet three times daily for 7 days.

10. Rx   Dipivefrin Hydrochloride
           0.1% Solution   20 mL
           Sig. For the eye.
    How many milligrams of dipivefrin hydrochloride should be used to prepare this prescription?
    a. 20 mg
    b. 10 mg
    c. 2 mg
    d. 12 mg

11. Which vitamin is usually given in conjunction with INH (Isoniazid)?
    a. B1
    b. B2
    c. B5
    d. B6

12. Which vitamin is usually given in conjuction with Methotrexate?
    a. B1
    b. B9
    c. B12
    d. B6

13. Which drug is not a PCN (penicillin) antiobiotic?
    a. Augmentin
    b. Amoxicillin
    c. Clarithromycin
    d. Ampicillin

14. Which drug is classified as a calcium-channel blocker?
    a. Verapamil
    b. Furosemide
    c. Flecanide
    d. Atenolol

15. The recommended dose of a medication is 80 mg/kg/day four times daily, how should a 195 lb patient be dosed?
    a. 7091 mg per day
    b. 1773 mg qid
    c. 7,091,000 mcg per day
    d. All of the above

16. Which patch is not a controlled drug substance schedule CII?
    a. Daytrana
    b. Vivelle Dot
    c. Fentanyl
    d. All of the above are CDS CII

17. How are otic drops administered?
    a. By mouth
    b. In the ear
    c. In the eye
    d. On the toenails or fingernails

18. Metformin 500 mg, 2 po bid. Which statement is false?
    a. The directions state to take two tablets by mouth twice daily.
    b. Metformin is used for type II diabetes.
    c. Common side effect is weight gain.
    d. A major contraindication with this medication is in patients with congestive heart failure.

19. Digoxin is classified as what type of drug?
    a. Calcium-channel blocker
    b. Beta blocker
    c. Cardiac glycoside
    d. Angiotensin II receptor antagonist

20. A formula for a mouth rinse contains 1/25% (w/v) of potassium choride. How many grams of potassium chloride should be used in preparing 30 liters of the mouth rinse?
    a. 2 gm
    b. 12 gm
    c. 5 gm
    d. 10 gm
21. Which drug is an H2 antagonist?
    a. Clonidine
    b. Famotidine
    c. Lansoprazole
    d. Loratidine
22. What symptom would an expectorant be used to treat?
    a. Watery eyes
    b. Nasal congestion
    c. Runny nose
    d. Chest congestion
23. What symptom would an antitussive be used to treat?
    a. Cough
    b. Chest congestion
    c. Nasal congestion
    d. Runny nose
24. Lisinopril/HCTZ, 1 po qd #30. Which statement is false?
    a. This drug is taken in the morning due to increased urination.
    b. This drug combination does not exist.
    c. Lisinopril is an ACE inhibitor.
    d. HCTZ is an abbreviation for hydrochlorothiazide which is a diuretic.
25. Loratidine is classified as a/an _____.
    a. H1 antagonist
    b. Analgesic
    c. Antypyretic
    d. Antitussive
26. Mobic 15 mg, i po q am qty 30. Which statement is false?
    a. Meloxicam is the generic name for Mobic.
    b. The directions state to take 1 tablet by mouth every morning.
    c. Mobic is a diuretic.
    d. Mobic is a NSAID.
27. What antidote is given to help increase blood clotting when an overdose of Heparin occurs?
    a. Vitamin B12
    b. Protamine
    c. Atropine
    d. Glucagon
28. What is the concentration of NS (normal saline)?
    a. 0.09% NaCl
    b. 0.9% NaCl
    c. 0.45% NaCl
    d. 0.045% NaCl
29. When will Augmentin suspension expire once it is reconstituted?
    a. 5 days
    b. 10 days
    c. 12 days
    d. 14 days

30. The intravenous dose of mannitol is 1.5 g/kg of body weight, administered as a 15 % (w/v) solution. How many milliliters of the solution should be administered to a 135 lb patient?
    a. 536 ml
    b. 214 ml
    c. 125 ml
    d. 614 ml

31. Actonel and Fosamax should be given at what time of the day?
    a. First thing in the morning
    b. Noon
    c. At bedtime
    d. It does not matter what time the drug is taken

32. A patient with chest congestion, cough and runny nose should be treated with which combination?
    a. Expectorant, proton pump inhibitor and an antihistamine
    b. Antitussive, antipyretic and an antiimflamitory
    c. Expectorant, antitussive and an antihistamine
    d. Antihistamine, antipyretic and an antitussive

33. A DEA 106 form is used _____.
    a. To order drugs
    b. To dispense drugs
    c. To report lost or stolen drugs
    d. To open a new pharmacy

34. Vicodin 5/500, i po prn pain. #120. Which statement is false?
    a. The directions state to take one tablet by mouth as needed for pain.
    b. This drug is a control drug substance CIII.
    c. This medication contains hydrocodone.
    d. The maximum daily dose of Acetaminophen is 6000 mg.

35. Which drug is not used to treat diabetes?
    a. Glipizide
    b. Metformin
    c. Rosiglitazone
    d. Avapro

36. A DEA 222 form is used _____.
    a. To order controlled drug substance schedule CII drugs
    b. To dispense controlled drug substance schedule CII drugs
    c. To report lost or stolen control drug substances
    d. To open a new pharmacy that will dispense control drug substances

37. Which antidote would be used to treat an overdose of APAP (acetaminophen)?
    a. Acetylcystine
    b. Narcan
    c. Naloxone
    d. Antabuse

38. Polytrim ophthalmic, V gtts os tid x 10d. Which statement is true?
    a. The directions state to instill 10 drops into left eye three times daily for 10 days.
    b. The abbreviation "os" means left eye.
    c. The abbreviation "os" means left ear.
    d. The abbreviation "os" means right ear.

39. A prescription calls for 240 ml of Lubriderm and 120 mg of kenalog. The kenalog vial has a concentration of 40 mg/ml. How much kenalog should be injected into the Lubriderm?
    a. 1 ml
    b. 2 ml
    c. 3 ml
    d. 4 ml

40. A pharmacist incorporates 10 gm of lidocaine into 150 gm of a 5% lidocaine ointment. Calculate the percentage (w/w) of lidocaine in the finished product.
    a.   2.5%
    b.   7.5%
    c.   5.2%
    d.   10.9%

41. If a patient is taking Atenolol, Accupril and Hydrochlorothiazide, which disease state is being treated?
    a.   Diabetes
    b.   Hypertension
    c.   Hyperlipidemia
    d.   Bacterial infection

42. Which drug would likely cause a dry cough?
    a.   Ramipril
    b.   Augmentin
    c.   Furosemide
    d.   Diltiazem

43. What is the correct way to clean a laminar flow hood?
    a.   Using sterile warm water only.
    b.   The laminar flow hood is self cleaning but must be swabbed for microbes every 6 months.
    c.   Disinfect with water and 70% isopropyl alcohol.
    d.   Any of the above will clean properly as long as it is cleaned and checked regularly.

44. Tobrex ophthalmic drops, i gtt ou bid x 7d. Which statement is false?
    a.   The directions state to instill one drop into each eye twice daily for 7 days.
    b.   Tobrex is an aminoglycoside antibiotic.
    c.   This should be instilled into each ear.
    d.   This should be instilled into each eye.

45. What is HIPAA's primary goal?
    a.   To protect a practitioner from law suits.
    b.   Allows Doctors and Pharmacies to distribute patient information as they deem necessary.
    c.   To protect patient's health information
    d.   States that a pharmacist must make an offer to counsel patients.

46. Which of the following drugs is vitamin B9?
    a.   Riboflavin
    b.   Niacin
    c.   Thiamine
    d.   Folic acid

47. Which of the following would be used to treat a type I diabetic?
    a.   Metformin
    b.   Lantus
    c.   Actos
    d.   Avandia

48. When counseling a patient taking a diuretic, they should know that it will cause _____.
    a.   Increased urination
    b.   Hair loss
    c.   Constipation
    d.   Discolored urine and feces.

49. Which drug is not a non-steroidal anti-inflammatory?
    a.   Ketoprofen
    b.   Ibuprofen
    c.   Naproxen
    d.   Tramadol

50. Which drug is not an antihistamine?
    a. Loratidine
    b. Clemestine
    c. Fexofenadine
    d. Sertraline

51. How many grams of 35% lidocaine ointment should be mixed with petrolatum to prepare 3 lbs of 5% lidocaine ointment?
    a. 195 gm of 35% lidocaine ointment
    b. 98 gm of 35% lidocaine ointment
    c. 236 gm of 35% lidocaine ointment
    d. 298 gm of 35% lidocaine ointment

52. To prevent flushing when taking niacin, what should a patient do?
    a. Take an aspirin 30 minutes prior to taking niacin
    b. Take niacin with meals
    c. Take niacin on an empty stomach
    d. Do not lie down for one hour after taking niacin

53. Tobradex (Tobramycin/Dexamethasone), i gtt od qid x 5d. Which statement is true?
    a. The directions state to take one drop by mouth every other day for 5 days.
    b. The directions state to instill one drop into left ear four times daily for 5 days.
    c. The directions state to instill one drop into left eye four times daily for 5 days.
    d. The directions state to instill one drop into right eye four times daily for 5 days.

54. What is the abbreviation for both eyes?
    a. au
    b. ou
    c. hs
    d. os

55. What is the abbreviation for after meals?
    a. ac
    b. pc
    c. hs
    d. dc

56. Methotrexate is usually dosed?
    a. Once daily
    b. Once weekly
    c. Once monthly
    d. None of the above

57. Which drug is not a pregnancy category "X" drug?
    a. Coumadin
    b. Pseudoephedrine
    c. Accutane
    d. Alcohol

58. Which category is absolutely safe to use during pregnancy?
    a. A
    b. B
    c. C
    d. D

59. How many grams of 5% (w/w) boric acid solution can be made from 1500 g of 50% (w/w) boric acid solution?
    a. 10,000 g
    b. 500 g
    c. 25,000 g
    d. 15,000 g

60. Which statement is false concerning H1 antagonist antihistamines?
    a. They treat allergies.
    b. They treat runny nose and watery eyes.
    c. Diphenhydramine is a H1 antagonist.
    d. Phenylepherine is a H1 antagonist.

61. Antitussives are used to treat _____.
    a. Gas
    b. Cough
    c. Itching
    d. Hiccups

62. Proton Pump Inhibitors help with which disease state?
    a. CHF (congestive heart failure)
    b. GERD (gastro esophageal reflux disease)
    c. HTN (hypertension)
    d. Gout

63. How many milliliters are in one pint?
    a. 480 ml
    b. 560 ml
    c. 240 ml
    d. 946 ml

64. One tablespoon contains how many milliliters?
    a. 5 ml
    b. 10 ml
    c. 15 ml
    d. 30 ml

65. Nitroglycerin is considered a/an _____.
    a. Antibiotic
    b. Vasoconstrictor
    c. Vasodilator
    d. Hyperlipidemic

66. Which drug is not considered a rapid acting insulin?
    a. Humalog (insulin Lispro)
    b. Apidra (insulin glulisine)
    c. Novolog (insulin asparte)
    d. Lantus (insulin glargine)

67. How much water should be mixed with 2500 ml of 75 % (v/v) alcohol to make 50 % (v/v) alcohol?
    a. 2000 ml
    b. 5000 ml
    c. 3750 ml
    d. 4000 ml

68. What situation would not require a child resistant container?
    a. Nitroglycerin sublingual tablets
    b. When a pharmacy in a hospital fills a prescription for an inpatient
    c. When a patient signs a child resistant disclaimer form
    d. All of the above

69. Which drug would not require a child resistant container?
    a. Albuterol syrup
    b. Nitroglycerin sublingual tablets
    c. Penicillin tablets
    d. None of the above require child resistant containers

70. What is the Orange Book's major objective?
    a. To give the therapeutic equivalency of drugs
    b. To give the cost of drugs
    c. To give the monographs of drugs
    d. To give the molecular structures of drugs

71. The primary benefit of a drug formulary in a hospital is to:
    a.   Allow doctors to have complete freedom of choice when prescribing medicines
    b.   Allow hospital to reduce inventory and therefore reduce cost
    c.   Allow for a quicker recovery time for its patients
    d.   Facilitate the processing of insurance claims

72. Which bioequivalency rating would allow a drug to be substituted for another?
    a.   A
    b.   B
    c.   C
    d.   D

73. The Orphan Drug Act:
    a.   Gives the FDA a list of drugs annually that need to be formulated
    b.   Allows for drugs to be made for a small percentage of the population
    c.   Explains how drugs may be recalled due to adverse reactions
    d.   Explains which drugs require special registeration in order to be dispensed

74. A DEA 106 form is used for?
    a.   Ordering any controlled drug substance
    b.   Ordering only controlled drug substance schedule CII drugs
    c.   Reporting lost or stolen controlled drug substances
    d.   Used when destroying controlled drug substances

75. What is the percentage strength (v/v) of alcohol in a mixture of 2000 mL of 35% (v/v) alcohol, 750 mL of 55% (v/v) alcohol, and 750 mL of 65% (v/v) alcohol?
    a.   33.2%
    b.   25.9%
    c.   45.7%
    d.   52.7%

76. NPO means _____.
    a.   No known allergies
    b.   Nothing by mouth
    c.   Opthalmic solution
    d.   Otic solution

77. What is the proper distance that should be worked inside a laminar flow hood?
    a.   2 inches
    b.   6 inches
    c.   12 inches
    d.   16 inches

78. What is the maximum amount of refills that are permitted on controlled drug substances CIII-CV?
    a.   1
    b.   5
    c.   None
    d.   Whatever the doctor writes for

79. How long is a legend drug prescription valid?
    a.   1 month
    b.   6 months
    c.   1 year
    d.   Until the doctor deactivates the prescription

80. What filter size would be considered a sterilizing filter?
    a.   0.22 micron
    b.   0.3 micron
    c.   0.9 micron
    d.   1.0 micron

81. A controlled drug substance is written for "prn" refills. How many refills would be allowed?
    a.   1
    b.   4
    c.   5
    d.   None of the above

82. Which of the following drugs would be considered an OTC product?
   a. Naproxen 500 mg
   b. Folic acid 1 mg
   c. Acetaminophen 650 mg
   d. Zocor 20 mg
83. "Ung" is the abbreviation for _____.
   a. Cream
   b. Ointment
   c. Solution
   d. Suspension
84. How many grams of 5% diphenhydramine cream should be mixed with 0.5% diphenhydramine cream to make 500 gm of 2% diphenhydramine cream?
   a. 87 gm of 5% diphenhydramine cream
   b. 167 gm of 5% diphenhydramine cream
   c. 227 gm of 5% diphenhydramine cream
   d. 422 gm of 5% diphenhydramine cream
85. Which of the following statements is true?
   a. Hoods should be serviced every 6 months
   b. Hood pre-filters should be cleaned or changed every month
   c. Clean hoods with 70% isopropyl alcohol and from back to front with a side-to-side motion
   d. All of the above
86. An IV bolus is given _____.
   a. All at once
   b. Over a short period of time
   c. Over a long period of time
   d. None of the above
87. What type of injection has the quickest onset of action?
   a. Intravenous
   b. Intramuscular
   c. Intradermal
   d. Subcutaneously
88. Sterile solutions:
   a. Contain no bacteria or viruses
   b. Contain a minimum amount of bacteria and viruses
   c. Are only given to immunosuppressed patients
   d. Are always cloudy
89. Eye drops can be given in the ear but ear drops cannot be given in the eye.
   a. True
   b. False
90. Rantidine is classified as a/an _____.
   a. Antitussive
   b. Antihistamine
   c. Expectorant
   d. Nasal decongestant
91. If a patient takes one teaspoonful of Benadryl every 6 hours, how many milliliters would be taken in a 24 hour period?
   a. 10 ml
   b. 20 ml
   c. 30 ml
   d. 40 ml
92. The core of a rubber closure can be carved out when _____.
   a. The needle is too large
   b. The needle is too small
   c. The needle is not removed from the vial properly
   d. The needle is inserted into the vial improperly

93. What is the generic name for Persantine?
    a. Dexamethasone
    b. Phenobarbital
    c. Dipyridamole
    d. Cyclobenazeprine
94. What government institution requires accurate drug accountability records for investigational drugs?
    a. DEA
    b. DPS
    c. OSHA
    d. FDA
95. How many milliliters of a 60% (w/v) sucrose solution and how many milliliters of 10% (w/v) sucrose solution are required to prepare 5000 mL of a 20 % solution?
    a. 1000ml 60%, 4000ml 10%
    b. 100ml 60%, 2000ml 10%
    c. 2000ml 60%, 3000ml 10%
    d. 4500ml 60%, 500ml 10%
96. What amount of Digoxin would be present in 2.5 ml of a 0.05mg/ml Digoxin elixir?
    a. 12.5 mcg
    b. 12.5 gm
    c. 125 mcg
    d. 0.0125 mg
97. What is the mechanism of action of Nitroglycerin?
    a. Angiotension II receptor antagonist
    b. Alpha blocker
    c. Vasodilator
    d. Vasoconstrictor
98. Rifampin is used as an _____.
    a. Anti-infective
    b. Anticonvulsant
    c. Antineoplastic
    d. Antimigraine
99. Angina would be described as:
    a. The heart receiving insufficient oxygen
    b. An embolism in the lung
    c. Light headedness upon suddenly standing
    d. An embolism in the brain
100. Which of the following would be classified as an anticoagulant?
    a. Vitamin K
    b. Nitroglycerin
    c. Warfarin
    d. Minoxidil
101. An Armour Thyroid prescription is written for 90 mg, this is equivalent to:
    a. 1/2 grain
    b. 1 grains
    c. 1 & 1/2 grains
    d. 2 grains
102. A prescription is written for Amoxil 500 mg every 12 hours for 10 days. The patient cannot take tablets and request a suspension. If the only available suspension in the pharmacy is 400mg/5 ml what would be the new sig?
    a. 2 teaspoonful every 12 hours
    b. 4.2 ml every 12 hours
    c. 1 tablespoonful every 12 hours
    d. 6.25 ml every 12 hours

103. Which of the following is not an antidepressant?
    a. Fluoxetine
    b. Elavil
    c. Zoloft
    d. Imitrex
104. The label of a dry powder for oral suspension states that when 98 mL of water are added to the powder, 150 mL of a suspension containing 300 mg of penicillin per 5 mL are prepared. How many milliliters of water should be used to prepare, in each 5 mL of product, the correct dose of penicillin for a 50 lb child based on the dose of 5 mg/kg of body weight?
    a. 300.5 ml
    b. 250 ml
    c. 405.5 ml
    d. 344.1 ml
105. A technician reads the temperature in the refrigerator as 62 degrees F. The refrigerator is _____.
    a. Too hot
    b. Too cold
    c. Just the right temperature
    d. It does not matter what the temperature of the refrigerator is as long as the medication stays cool.
106. According to federal law, a perpetual inventory must be kept on which controlled drug substance schedule?
    a. Schedule I
    b. Schedule II
    c. Schedule III
    d. Schedule V
107. Which drug is not a controlled drug substance?
    a. Lomotil
    b. Oxycodone
    c. Xanax
    d. Clonidine
108. Teratogenic is a term that means _____.
    a. May cause birth defects
    b. Medication should not be taken if patient is under 18 years old
    c. May cause heart problems
    d. May cause loss of hearing
109. A satellite pharmacy in a hospital, which allows for quicker delivery of medication, is known as a
_____.
    a. Decentralized pharmacy
    b. Independent pharmacy
    c. Category A pharmacy
    d. Category C pharmacy
110. If a net profit is realized by the pharmacy it could be said that?
    a. The pharmacy is losing money
    b. Revenues are greater than total expenses
    c. Inventory turnover is slow
    d. Expenses are greater than cost of goods sold
111. A vertical flow hood would be needed to prepare which of the following?
    a. Mefoxin 2 gm in D5W 100 ml
    b. Clindamyin 900 mg in D5W 100 ml
    c. Vincristine 5 mg in NS 100 ml
    d. Vancomycin 1 gm in NS 250 ml

112. What information will the manufacturers give the pharmacy when notifying them of a drug recall to ensure only the drugs affected will be pulled and sent back?
   a. AWP of the drug
   b. UPC number
   c. Lot number
   d. Strength of drug

113. How many gallons of promethzine with codeine would be in 144 pints?
   a. 10 gallons
   b. 14 gallons
   c. 18 gallons
   d. 20 gallons

114. A prescription reading Promethazine 25 mg 1q6h for 3 days qty 12. What information is missing?
   a. Diagnosis code
   b. Route of administration
   c. Indication
   d. Duration

115. A patient is taking maintenance Naproxen and is about to have major surgery. What is a very important piece of information that the patient should be counseled on?
   a. Continue taking medication to keep a steady state level in the body
   b. There is no problem taking Naproxen prior to a major surgery
   c. Oral Naproxen is incompatible with most IV medications and therefore should be discontinued prior to surgery
   d. Naproxen should be discontinued prior to a major surgery due to the blood thinning properties of Naproxen

116. A med guide is mandatory when dispensing which of the following drugs?
   a. Diazepam
   b. Amoxil
   c. Ketoprofen
   d. Fexofenadine

117. Which would be written on a prescription to designate that the drug should be taken after meals?
   a. p.o.
   b. h.s.
   c. p.c.
   d. prn

118. 2 degrees C to 8 degrees C (36 degrees F to 46 degrees F) refers to which temperature?
   a. Refrigerated
   b. Cool
   c. Room temperature
   d. Frozen

119. The generic name for Restoril is _____.
   a. Temazpepam
   b. Diazepam
   c. Lorazepam
   d. Clonazepam

120. Pravastatin is used to treat _____.
   a. Hyperlipidemia
   b. Hypertension
   c. Angina
   d. Leg cramps

121. A prescription reads:
   Kenalog 60 mg mixed in 240 g of Lubriderm
   How much kenalog will need to be drawn up if Kenalog comes in a 40mg/ml vial?
   a. 0.5 ml
   b. 1 ml
   c. 1.5 ml
   d. 2 ml.

122. A patient weighs 37 lbs. The physician orders state to give 15mg/kg/day divided every 12 hours for 10 days.
    I. How much does the patient weigh in Kg?
        a. 16.8 kg
        b. 22 kg
        c. 81.4 kg
        d. 59.4 kg
    II. How many mg/day will be given?
        a. 187 mg
        b. 252 mg
        c. 384 mg
        d. 96 mg
    III. What will be the total dose given over the 10 day period?
        a. 1860
        b. 2634
        c. 2522
        d. 3256

123. The following prescription is given to the pharmacy technician:
    Lortab elixir 8 oz.
    1 tsp po q 4 h prn
Which auxiliary label would be placed on the prescription bottle?
    a. May cause diarrhea
    b. May cause drowsiness
    c. Keep refrigerated
    d. For external use only

124. The following prescription is written:
    Zantac 75mg/5ml
    1 teaspoonful by mouth every day
How many ml will be given in one month?
    a. 150 ml
    b. 120 ml
    c. 180 ml
    d. 200 ml

125. The greatest benefit of packaging medication in a unit dose package from a bulk supply is:
    a. Reducing the time it takes the technician to count medication
    b. Makes it easier for pharmacist to view medication
    c. Decreases pharmacist chance of making an error
    d. Makes pharmacy more organized

126. The middle four NDC numbers represent _____.
    a. The quantity
    b. The manufacturer
    c. The product
    d. The dosage form

127. Which medication should be protected from light?
    a. Nitroprusside
    b. Ranitidine
    c. Sumitriptan
    d. Risperdal

128. Methamphetamine would be classified in which controlled drug substance schedule?
    a. CI
    b. CII
    c. CIII
    d. CIV

129. Which of the following drugs is not a controlled substance?
- a. Daytrana
- b. Flexeril
- c. Lomotil
- d. Halcion

130. Which of the following is required to be on a controlled drug substance schedule CII prescription?
- a. Doctors DEA number
- b. Patients name
- c. Date the prescription was written
- d. All of the above

131. How long must a DEA 222 form be kept on file?
- a. 1 year
- b. 2 years
- c. 5 years
- d. 10 years

132. A DEA 222 form is used to order _____.
- a. All controlled substances
- b. Only narcotic controlled substances
- c. All controlled drug substance schedule CII drugs
- d. All controlled drug substance schedule CI and CII drugs

133. Ipecac syrup is used to _____.
- a. Induce vomiting
- b. Relieve constipation
- c. Alleviate nausea
- d. Is an antidote for acetaminophen poisoning

134. Which of the following is not a controlled drug substance schedule CI?
- a. Peyote
- b. Heroin
- c. Cocaine
- d. All of the above are controlled drug substance schedule CI's

135. What is the maximum amount of Ipecac syrup that can be sold without a prescription?
- a. 15 ml
- b. 30 ml
- c. 45 ml
- d. There is no maximum amount that can be purchased

136. Drugs that are "Grandfathered" are drugs that were marketed before the passage of?
- a. Durham-Humphrey Act
- b. Food, Drug and Cosmetic Act of 1938
- c. Poison Prevention Act of 1970
- d. Harrison Narcotic Act of 1914

137. Which of the following drugs is not a cephalosporin?
- a. Cefprozil
- b. Keflex
- c. Cefixime
- d. Coreg

138. What amount of 100% lanolin ointment must be diluted with white petrolatum to fill an order for 1/2 pound of 15% lanolin ointment? [Assume 1 lb = 454 g]
- a. 23 gm
- b. 39 gm
- c. 34 gm
- d. 19 gm

139. Which of the following is not a barbiturate?
- a. Pentobarbital
- b. Methohexital
- c. Phenobarbital
- d. Dicyclomine

140. You have an order for a solution of 2% dextrose in NS to be given in a 5 hour IV infusion. The Pharmacy has a 500 ml IV bag of saline and a 40% dextrose solution in stock. What volume of the 40% solution should be added to the IV bag?
    a. 25 ml
    b. 250 ml
    c. 10 ml
    d. 20 ml

141. Which of the following is an antipyretic?
    a. Naproxen
    b. Digoxin
    c. Acyclovir
    d. Bisoprolol

142. A patient is taking three 600 mg capsules of lithium each day. How many mg of lithium would the patient take in 30 days?
    a. 26,000 mg
    b. 34,000 mg
    c. 54,000 mg
    d. 62,000 mg

143. An IV infusion order is received for piperacillin-tazobactam (Zosyn) 3.375 g in 500 mL of NS to be infused at 113 mg/min. What will the flow rate be in mL/hr?
    a. 435.6 ml/hr
    b. 1400.3 ml/hr
    c. 988.5 ml/hr
    d. 1004.4 ml/hr

144. An IV infusion order is received for furosemide (Lasix) 40 mg in 500 mL of NS, to be infused at 75 mL/hr. What amount of furosemide will the patient receive per hour?
    a. 6 mg/hr
    b. 3 mg/hr
    c. 9 mg/hr
    d. 10 mg/hr

145. Dilantin is to Phenytoin as Zoloft is to:
    a. Sertaline
    b. Simvastatin
    c. Zymar
    d. Alprazolam

146. A 500 ml bag of 0.25% NS runs at 60 gtt/min with an infusion delivering 10 gtt/ml. How long will the infusion last?
    a. 3.6 hours
    b. 1.39 hours
    c. 2.9 hour
    d. 4.2 hours

147. Where on a graduated cylinder should the volume of an aqueous liquid be read?
    a. Top of the liquid
    b. Volume drawn into a syringe
    c. Bottom of the meniscus
    d. Top of the meniscus

148. The Pharmacy and Therapeutics (P&T) committee's primary function is?
    a. Create credentialing requirements for pharmacy employees
    b. Regulate the therapeutic use of pharmaceutical products
    c. Enforce state pharmacy laws and FDA regulations
    d. Provide therapy to the pharmacy community

149. If 20 gallons of distilled water cost $45.25, how much will 5 gallons cost?
    a. $11.31
    b. $14.75
    c. $19.25
    d. $8.79

150. An order asks for amoxicillin 250 mg BID for 10 days. If a 100 mg/5 mL suspension is used, what will the volume of each dose be?
   a. 5 ml
   b. 7.5 ml
   c. 12.5 ml
   d. 2.5 ml

Practice Test #3

1. A bottle of Atenolol has a expiration date of 10/2006. What day will the drug expire?
    a. 9/30/2006
    b. 10/01/2006
    c. 10/31/2006
    d. 11/01/2006

2. When dispensing birth control tablets, how often must a package insert be included?
    a. Only when the original prescription is dipensed
    b. Once yearly
    c. Every time the prescription is filled
    d. Birth control is not a prescription that needs a package insert dispensed with the prescription.

3. Psuedoephedrine would be contraindicated in a patient taking which medication?
    a. Simvastatin
    b. Levaquin
    c. Nifedipine
    d. Zolpidem

4. Which drug is used for hyperthyroidism?
    a. Levoxyl
    b. Cytomel
    c. Propylthiouracil
    d. Armour thyroid

5. Which of the following is not a dosage form of clonidine?
    a. Transdermal patch
    b. Oral tablets
    c. Sublingual tablets
    d. Clonidine comes in all of the above dosage forms

6. If 0.025 gm thyroid extract contains 50 mcg of levothyroxine, how much levothyroxine is contained in 2.5 mg of thyroid extract?
    a. 5 mcg
    b. 7.5 mcg
    c. 12.5 mcg
    d. 10 mcg

7. A pharmacy technician wants to add 75 mg of a particular drug to 100 mL of NS. The drug solution is supplied in a 2% concentration. What is the volume of the 2% concentration required to supply 75 mg of the drug?
    a. 2 ml
    b. 5 ml
    c. 3.75 ml
    d. 7.5 ml

8. A 66-lb child is given a prescription for Amoxicillin. The recommended child dose is 25 mg/kg/day in two doses. What is the correct dose to be given?
    a. 259 mg
    b. 623 mg
    c. 325 mg
    d. 375 mg

9. A prescription reads "2 tsp q 4 -6h 10d". How much medication should be dispensed?
    a. 60 tablets
    b. 400 ml
    c. 600 ml
    d. 40 tablets

10. An otic preparation would be placed in the:
    a. Ear
    b. Eyes
    c. Mouth
    d. Nose

11. The last two numbers of an NDC number represent which of the following?
    a. Manufacturer
    b. Unit package size
    c. Product strength
    d. Dosage form
12. On an order for Dilantin 100 mg capsules #XXX, what would be the correct quantity to dispense?
    a. 300 capsules
    b. 3 capsules
    c. 30 capsules
    d. 100 capules
13. What volume of a digoxin concentration 0.25mg/5ml will deliver a dose of 0.250mg?
    a. 10 ml
    b. 5 ml
    c. 15 ml
    d. 20 ml
14. A pharmacy fills an order for #30 Cipro tablets containing 0.250 gm of ciprofloxacin each. What are the total milligrams of ciprofloxacin dispensed?
    a. 5000 mg
    b. 7500 mg
    c. 2200 mg
    d. 1800 mg
15. How many milliliters of ciprofloxacin suspension (250 mg/5 mL) would be needed to fill a prescription for ciprofloxacin 500 mg PO q12h for 10 days?
    a. 50 ml
    b. 250 ml
    c. 150 ml
    d. 200 ml
16. A liquid contains 0.5 mg/mL of a substance. How much of the substance will 4.2 L contain?
    a. 2100 mg
    b. 1000 mg
    c. 1400 mg
    d. 2500 mg
17. A prescription order specifies potassium chloride 20 mEq po BID. What volume of KCl solution containing 20 mEq/15 mL will be required to deliver a single dose?
    a. 5 ml
    b. 7.5 ml
    c. 15 ml
    d. 20 ml
18. Sublingual refers to giving a drug by:
    a. Swallowing it
    b. Placing it under the tongue
    c. Placing it in the cheek
    d. Inserting it rectally
19. When measuring 8 ml of a liquid, which size beaker should be used?
    a. 5 ml beaker
    b. 10 ml beaker
    c. 15 ml beaker
    d. 20 ml beaker
20. Which antibiotic would be the best choice for a patient that is allergic to cephalosporins?
    a. Augmentin
    b. Keflex
    c. Cefprozil
    d. Azithromycin

21. Which drug is not considered to be a pregnancy category "X" drug?
    a. Pseudoephedrine
    b. Coumadin
    c. Accutane
    d. Zocor
22. Which of the following drugs is a benzodiazepine?
    a. Klonopin
    b. Lorazepam
    c. Chlordiazepoxide
    d. All of the above
23. Photosensitivity can be seen when using which of the following medications?
    a. Cipro
    b. Gatifloxacin
    c. Tetracycline
    d. All of the above
24. Which of the following drugs can be used in young children?
    a. Tetracycline
    b. Ciprofloxacin
    c. Levaquin
    d. None of the above
25. Once reconstituted, refrigerated augmentin suspension is stable for how many days?
    a. 5 days
    b. 10 days
    c. 14 days
    d. 20 days
26. If 200 tablets contain 400 mg of a substance, how many grains would 600 tablets contain?
    a. 6 grn
    b. 10 grn
    c. 20 grn
    d. 24 grn
27. The metric equivalent of a 5 grain dose of Aspirin is:
    a. 81 mg
    b. 150 mg
    c. 325 mg
    d. 650 mg
28. If 2 kg of a cream contains 500 g of triamcinolone, what is the percentage strength of the cream?
    a. 25%
    b. 12%
    c. 33%
    d. 7%
29. Which of the following drugs causes a yellow discoloration of the urine?
    a. Penicillin
    b. Cephalexin
    c. Vitamin B2 (riboflavin)
    d. Alprazolam
30. Which of the following drugs causes a reddish-brown discoloration of the urine?
    a. Phenazopyridine
    b. Diphenhydramine
    c. Amoxicillin
    d. Propranolol
31. What volume of Pepto Bismol would be dispensed to administer a dose of 2 oz?
    a. 30 ml
    b. 60 ml
    c. 80 ml
    d. 15 ml

32. A cash discount of $250 on a pharmacy invoice for $7700 represents a percentage cash discount of:
    a. 5%
    b. 3.25%
    c. 1.25%
    d. 7.5%

33. A 40 mL dose of a mixture prescribed for pain relief contains 30 mg codeine, 325 mg acetaminophen, 10 mL grape syrup q.s. with water. How many 60 mg codeine tables are needed to prepare 480 mL of this solution?
    a. 2
    b. 8
    c. 6
    d. 12

34. Which route of administration should Floxin otic drops be given?
    a. By mouth
    b. In the ear
    c. In the eye
    d. Intranasally

35. How far inside a laminar flow hood should a technician work?
    a. 4 inches inside the hood
    b. As far inside the hood as possible
    c. Anywhere, as long as medication is being prepared inside the hood
    d. At least 6 inches inside the hood

36. How many times may a prescription of methadone be refilled?
    a. Five times
    b. Six times
    c. One time
    d. Cannot be refilled

37. Which pregnancy category shows no risk in pregnancy?
    a. A
    b. B
    c. C
    d. D

38. "Statins" (HMG-CoA reductase inhibitors) are used to treat which disease state?
    a. Hypertension
    b. Migraine headaches
    c. Hyperlipidemia
    d. Antifungal

39. Which two drug classes have cross sensitivity?
    a. Fluoroquinolones and Tetracyclines
    b. Sulfonamides and Penicillins
    c. Macrolides and Aminoglycosides
    d. Penicillins and Cephalosporins

40. The process by which is a drug is broken down in the body is called?
    a. Metabolism
    b. Absorption
    c. Titration
    d. Elimination

41. A prescription reads: Omnicef 250mg/5ml, 1 tsp po qd x 10 days. How many milliliters of Omnicef will be given over the 10 days?
    a. 25 ml
    b. 50 ml
    c. 75 ml
    d. 100 ml

42. What type of solution is recommended when cleaning a laminar flow hood?
    a. A mixture of 10:1 water and bleach
    b. 70% Isopropyl alcohol
    c. An isotonic solution
    d. Warm soapy water
43. Which type of insulin may be added to an IV solution?
    a. Glargine
    b. 70/30 mix
    c. Regular
    d. No type of insulin should be added to a IV
44. Which drug would not be used to treat elevated cholesterol and/or triglycerides?
    a. Pravachol
    b. Niacin
    c. Atenolol
    d. Zetia
45. A prescription has directions that read: 1 gtt od qid x 5 days. What does "od" mean?
    a. Right ear
    b. Left ear
    c. Right eye
    d. Left eye
46. A prescription has directions that read: 2 gtt ou tid x 10 days. What does "ou' mean?
    a. Left eye
    b. Both eyes
    c. Right ear
    d. Both ears
47. A patient is to be administered a drug that has a recommended dosage of 2 mg/kg of body weight. The patient is a child weighing 40 lbs. What amount of the drug should the patient receive?
    a. 24.2 mg
    b. 36.4 mg
    c. 43.1 mg
    d. 54.6 mg
48. How much nystatin must be added to triamcinolone cream to dispense an order for 60 g of triamcinolone cream with 2% nystatin?
    a. 0.5 g
    b. 5 g
    c. 3.5 g
    d. 1.2 g
49. A prescription requires a 50 mg dose of IV Diazepam, and the pharmacy only stocks vials of Diazepam 10 mg/mL. What volume of this solution will be required to dispense the correct dose?
    a. 5ml
    b. 10ml
    c. 3ml
    d. 15ml
50. How many 875 mg Amoxicillin tablets are required to prepare 1000 mL of a 250 mg/ 5 mL concentration?
    a. 24
    b. 58
    c. 12
    d. 67
51. Which of the following drugs would not be considered to be an antidepressant?
    a. Citalopram
    b. Sertraline
    c. Trazodone
    d. Lidoderm

52. How many milliliters are in one pint?
    a. 120 ml
    b. 240 ml
    c. 480 ml
    d. 960 ml
53. Which drug would have an auxiliary label reading "May Discolor Urine"?
    a. Ciprofloxicn
    b. Etodolac
    c. Allopurinol
    d. Pyridium
54. What would be the most appropriate attire to wear when working with chemotherapeutic drugs?
    a. Normal dress clothes
    b. Goggles and a hair net
    c. Gloves and goggles
    d. Full body covering including gloves, hair covering and a mask
55. How many milliliters are in two and three-fourths teaspoonful?
    a. 7.5 ml
    b. 10.5 ml
    c. 13.75 ml
    d. 17.5 ml
56. Diphenhydramine:
    a. Comes in both a cream and a tablet
    b. Is an antihistamine
    c. Can be used for itching
    d. All of the above
57. Which statement regarding a cloudy IV bag is true?
    a. Should be discarded
    b. A cloudy IV bag is acceptable only if used within 12 hours
    c. A cloudy TPN IV admixture is acceptable
    d. A cloudy IV bag is acceptable only if used within 6 hours
58. Which of the following is not an NSAID?
    a. Ketoprofen
    b. Naproxen
    c. Motrin
    d. Acetaminophen
59. Which is true concerning the gauge size of a needle?
    a. The higher the gauge the thinner the needle
    b. The higher the gauge the thicker the needle
    c. The higher the gauge the longer the needle
    d. The higher the gauge the shorter the needle
60. A Heparin drip is given at a concentration of 25 units/mL and dosed at 1000 units/hr. How many mL/hr would be given to the patient?
    a. 40 ml/hr
    b. 20 ml/hr
    c. 10 ml/hr
    d. 25 ml/hr
61. How many grams of Dextrose are contained in a 5 mL solution of Dextrose 25%?
    a. 5 gm
    b. 10 gm
    c. 1.25 gm
    d. 2.5 gm

62. What volume of 3 mEq/mL NaCl injection must be added to a TPN solution to deliver 40 mEq of NaCl?
    a. 13.33 ml
    b. 9.9 ml
    c. 16.9 ml
    d. 20 ml
63. A patient using 33 units of insulin every morning would require which size syringe?
    a. 0.3 cc
    b. 0.5 cc
    c. 1.0 cc
    d. 2.0 cc
64. Which government agency would be responsible for initiating a recall?
    a. DEA
    b. FDA
    c. OSHA
    d. DPS
65. If a patient had an anaphylactic reaction while taking acetaminophen, which drug could the patient take for pain?
    a. Percocet
    b. Ultram
    c. Vicodin
    d. Ultracet
66. A prescription reads: 1 po tid x 10 days. How many tablets should the patient receive?
    a. 10
    b. 20
    c. 30
    d. 40
67. How should a patient taking Flagyl be counseled?
    a. Take with food
    b. Do not drive, may cause drowsiness
    c. Do not drink alcohol
    d. May cause syncope
68. A meniscus is _____.
    a. A type of beaker
    b. A line of measurement
    c. A type of gelatin capsule
    d. A type of syringe
69. A list of drugs that an institution finds to be the most cost-effective and efficacious is called a _____.
    a. Inventory
    b. Formulary
    c. Profit and loss statement
    d. Compliance report
70. A prescription reads: 1 po tid pc and hs. The directions state:
    a. Take one by mouth twice daily before meals and after meals
    b. Take one by mouth three times daily before meals and at bedtime
    c. Take one by mouth four times daily after meals with food
    d. Take one by mouth three times daily after meals and at bedtime
71. Lasix should be taken _____.
    a. With food
    b. In the morning
    c. On an empty stomach
    d. Not with any other medications

72. Which strength is not commercially available?
    a. Fosamax 70 mg
    b. Lasix 80 mg
    c. Synthroid 5 mcg
    d. Zoloft 50 mg

73. A recommended dose of a drug is 30 mg/kg/day. How much of the drug should be administered to a patient weighing 75 kg?
    a. 1500 mg/day
    b. 2250 mg/day
    c. 2750 mg/day
    d. 1250 mg/day

74. What dosage will be delivered by an infusion of 500 mL of an IV solution containing 0.5 mg/mL of a medication?
    a. 250 mg
    b. 150 mg
    c. 350 mg
    d. 500 mg

75. A child is to receive Amoxicillin 40 mg/kg/day in equally divided doses every 8 hours. Which of the following manufacturer's product sizes should be used to reconstitute a 10 day supply for an 80 lb child if the label reads 400 mg/5 mL?
    a. 50 ml
    b. 300 ml
    c. 150 ml
    d. 200 ml

76. Which of the following drugs is not an antidepressant?
    a. Trazodone
    b. Celexa
    c. Lunesta
    d. Elavil

77. Which of the following drugs is not used for hypertension?
    a. Glucotrol
    b. Atenolol
    c. Quinipril
    d. Norvasc

78. Which of the following drugs is not an NSAID?
    a. Indocin
    b. Orudis
    c. Toradol
    d. Tramadol

79. Which of the following drugs is not a muscle relaxant?
    a. Baclofen
    b. Amiodarone
    c. Cyclobenaziprine
    d. Soma

80. A patient taking Coumadin can also take which of the following drugs without an adverse effect?
    a. Acetaminophen
    b. Aspirin
    c. Naproxen
    d. Ibuprofen

81. Which of the following drugs requires a package insert to be given when dispensing?
    a. Imdur
    b. Premarin
    c. Accupril
    d. Lyrica

82. A potassium supplement is commonly given in combination with which of the following drugs?
   - a. Soma
   - b. Lasix
   - c. Diabeta
   - d. Ziac
83. Which of the following drugs is available as a suspension?
   - a. Amoxil
   - b. Metoclopramide
   - c. Zyrtec
   - d. Zantac
84. Which one of the following drugs would not require a patient package insert?
   - a. Accutane
   - b. Cenestin
   - c. Norethindrone
   - d. Omeprazole
85. What do the first five, middle four and last two digits of a NDC number stand for?
   - a. Manufacturer, package size and drug
   - b. Manufacturer, drug and package size
   - c. Drug, package size and manufacturer
   - d. Package size, drug and manufacturer
86. A list of drug package inserts could be located in which one of the following books?
   - a. Fact and comparison
   - b. Drug topics
   - c. Physician desk reference
   - d. Orange book
87. 112 ml is equivalent to how many fluid ounces?
   - a. 1.2
   - b. 4.56
   - c. 2.44
   - d. 3.73
88. 150 grams is equivalent to how many mg?
   - a. 15,000 mg
   - b. 1500 mg
   - c. 150,000 mg
   - d. 150 mg
89. A doctor wants to give a patient 95 mg of Zantac 75mg/5ml. How many milliliters would need to be dispensed?
   - a. 6.3 ml
   - b. 5.0 ml
   - c. 13.0 ml
   - d. 8.9 ml
90. Subcutaneous injections are given _____.
   - a. Deep in the muscle
   - b. Directly under the skin
   - c. Directly in the vein
   - d. Through an IV
91. Which of the following diabetic injections is not an insulin?
   - a. Regular
   - b. Byetta
   - c. Lantus
   - d. Humalog
92. Hypoglycemia describes a condition in which:
   - a. There is too much thyroid hormone
   - b. Blood sugar is low
   - c. Cortisol level is too high
   - d. White blood cell count is low

93. How is oral penicillin usually taken?
    a. With food
    b. On an empty stomach
    c. Taken at night
    d. Once daily
94. When counseling a patient on antibiotics which statement is false?
    a. A patient should take all of the medication even if they are feeling better
    b. Counsel the patient to use another form of contraceptive if they are sexually active and taking oral birth control pills
    c. A female patient may consider taking Acidophilus to prevent a yeast infection
    d. All of the above are correct
95. Concerning intravenous solutions, which statement is false?
    a. It is given directly into the vein
    b. Aseptic techniques must be used in preparation of IV solutions
    c. It is always given in the left arm because it is closest to the heart
    d. It has a very rapid onset of action
96. IV bolus:
    a. Is given slowly over a long period of time
    b. Is given all at once
    c. Describes a type of piggyback technique
    d. All of the above are correct
97. An inventory system that maintains a continuous record of certain items is referred to as:
    a. Closed formulary
    b. Open formulary
    c. Perpetual inventory
    d. Dynamic inventory
98. How much Ceclor 250 mg per 2.5 ml suspension should be dispensed for a 350 mg dose?
    a. 2.5 ml
    b. 7.5 ml
    c. 3.5 ml
    d 9 ml
99. What volume of a 100 mg/ml injectable should be drawn up for 120 mg dose?
    a. 0.5 ml
    b. 1 ml
    c. 12 ml
    d. 1.2 ml
100. Which of the following statement is false?
    a. Aseptic technique must always be used when preparing IV solutions
    b. Discoloration of an IV bag is normal due to the mixing of different medications
    c. TPN preparations may be cloudy
    d. A equal volume of air should be injected into a vial that would equal the volume being removed to prevent a vacuum
101. Intramuscular injections:
    a. Use a larger needle than subcutaneous injections
    b. Can be used for vitamin B12 administration
    c. Are injected deeper than intradermal
    d. All of the above are correct
102. Which of the following statements is false?
    a. Horizontal hoods blow air through a filter towards the technician
    b. Vertical hoods blow air straight down to the work surface
    c. A hood should be turned on for at least 10 minutes before using
    d. All work must be done at least 6 inches inside the hood work surface

103. Which of the following drugs is not stored in the refrigerator?
    a. Combipatch
    b. Cardizem injection
    c. Xalatan
    d. Catapress patch
104. Which of the following statements is false?
    a. Hood pre-filters should be cleaned every month
    b. Hoods should be serviced once yearly
    c. Clean hoods with 70% isopropyl alcohol
    d. Hoods should be cleaned from back to front with a side-to-side motion
105. Controlled room temperature is _____.
    a. 20 to 25 degrees celcius or 68 to 77 degrees Fahrenheit
    b. 2 to 8 degrees celcius or 36 to 46 degrees Fahrenheit
    c. 10 to 15 degrees celcius or 54 to 68 degrees Fahrenheit
    d. None of the above are correct
106. Naloxone (Narcan) is an antidote for _____.
    a. Hypoglycemia
    b. Opiates
    c. Snake bites
    d. Mushrooms
107. Nitrostat 1/400 grains is equivalent to how many milligrams?
    a. 0.15 mg
    b. 0.4 mg
    c. 0.3 mg
    d. 0.6 mg
108. How many 100 mg doses are contained in 15 g of Cephalexin?
    a. 15
    b. 10
    c. 100
    d. 150
109. A 600 tablet bottle of ferrous sulfate cost $105.00. What would 150 tablets cost?
    a. $12.50
    b. $22.50
    c. $44.25
    d. $26.25
110. A 350 tablet bottle of ferrous sulfate cost $9.50. What would 35 tablets cost?
    a. $0.95
    b. $4.50
    c. $6.75
    d. $3.25
111. Flumazenil (Romazicon) is an antidote for _____.
    a. Acetaminophen
    b. Heparin
    c. Methotrexate
    d. Benzodiazepines
112. LX is a roman numeral that indicates which number?
    a. 20
    b. 60
    c. 35
    d. 90
113. Which of the following drugs is not an antibiotic?
    a. Avelox
    b. Vibramycin
    c. Rocephin
    d. Avandia

114. Which of the following drugs is not an antituberculosis drug?
    a.   Acyclovir
    b.   Isoniazid
    c.   Rifampin
    d.   Ethambutol

115. Which of the following drugs is not an antifungal?
    a.   Zovirax
    b.   Nystatin
    c.   Ketoconazole
    d.   Terbinafine

116. The Vioxx recall was an example of which type of recall?
    a.   Class I
    b.   Class II
    c.   Class III
    d.   Class IV

117. The cost of 1000 tablets of Ibuprofen 200 mg is $50.99. If a pharmacy markups the cost of the Ibupofen by 10%, what would be the retail charge for 50 tablets?
    a. $1.50
    b. $2.80
    c. $7.30
    d. $5.25

118. Which of the following drugs is not an antihistamine?
    a.   Fexofenadine
    b.   Chlorpheneramine
    c.   Sertraline
    d.   Zyrtec

119. Which controlled drug substance schedule would have the least potential for abuse?
    a.   Schedule I
    b.   Schedule II
    c.   Schedule III
    d.   Schedule IV
    e.   Schedule V

120. Which statement is false about a lozenge?
    a.   Should be swallowed immediately
    b.   A solid dosage form that slowly dissolves in the mouth
    c.   Also known as troches
    d.   Is usually flavored

121. Zantac comes in which dosage forms?
    a.   Tablet
    b.   Injection
    c.   Syrup
    d.   All of the above

122. A patient has an allergy to sulfur based drugs. Which drug would be contraindicated for this patient?
    a.   Bactrim
    b.   Augmentin
    c.   Mobic
    d.   Zoloft

123. A suppository is used in which route of administration?
    a.   Orally
    b.   Intranasally
    c.   Rectally
    d.   Topically

124. A sig reads 1 tablespoonful by mouth qid for 10 days. How many milliliters will be given daily?
    a. 20 ml
    b. 40 ml
    c. 60 ml
    d. 80 ml
125. A patient weighs 54 pounds how many kilograms does the patient weigh?
    a. 24 kg
    b. 118 kg
    c. 56 kg
    d. 88 kg
126. Which of the following drugs would be considered a local anesthetic?
    a. Benzocaine
    b. Lidocaine
    c. Xylocaine®
    d. All of the above
127. The AWP for a drug $ 65.99 with a 10% discount from the wholesaler. What would be the cost of this drug?
    a. $6.59
    b. $59.39
    c. $64.99
    d. $6.60
128. The AWP for a drug $ 26.99 with a 5% discount from the wholesaler. What would be the cost of this drug?
    a. $25.64
    b. $23.79
    c. $21.39
    d. $18.54
129. How many grams of a 2% hydrocortisone cream can be made from 350 grams of 4% cream?
    a. 350 g
    b. 1200 g
    c. 700 g
    d. 400 g
130. How much of 50% ethanol must be mixed with 25% ethanol to make 1 pint of 35% ethanol solution?
    a. 125 ml
    b. 192 ml
    c. 429 ml
    d. 288 ml
131. If a dose of Cephalexin is 34 mg/kg/day and the patient weighs 54 lbs. How many milligrams will be given daily?
    a. 400 mg
    b. 656 mg
    c. 833 mg
    d. 994 mg
132. Which combination of drugs would be considered duplicate therapy?
    a. Acetaminophen and Ibuprofen
    b. Avandia and Actos
    c. Atenolol and Norvasc
    d. Vicodin and Flexeril
133. A sig reads: 1 gtt os bid. Which statement is correct?
    a. One drop into left eye twice daily
    b. One drop into each ear twice daily
    c. One drop into right ear three times daily
    d. One drop into both eyes twice daily

134. Which of the following drugs does not contain Acetaminophen?
   a. Darvocet
   b. Vicodin
   c. Soma
   d. Percocet

135. Which auxiliary label should be attached on a prescription for Bactrim?
   a. Take with plenty of water
   b. May cause photosensitivity
   c. Finish all medication
   d. All of the above

136. A solution is described as:
   a. A mixture of water and alcohol
   b. A water and oil mixture
   c. A highly concentrated mixture of sugar, water, and alcohol
   d. Active ingredients are uniformly dispersed throughout the mixture.

137. Determine the flow rate of an IV if 125 ml of drug is to be infused over 2 hours. The administration set delivers 60 gtts/ml.
   a. 23gtts/min
   b. 63gtts/min
   c. 45gtts/min
   d. 77gtts/min

138. Determine the flow rate of an IVPB containing 150 ml of gentamycin. The solution is to be infused over a 1 hour period and the administration set is calibrated to deliver 10 drops per ml.
   a. 12 gtts/min
   b. 35 gtts/min
   c. 20 gtts/min
   d. 25 gtts/min

139. Which of the following antibiotics should be taken with an increased intake of water?
   a. Cefadroxil
   b. Azithromycin
   c. Sulfamethoxazole/Trimethoprim
   d. Minocycline

140. Which auxiliary label should be attached on a prescription for metronidazole?
   a. Take with plenty of water
   b. Avoid alcohol
   c. Shake well
   d. Wash hands after using

141. Which of the following drugs is used to treat tuberculosis?
   a. Acyclovir
   b. Cefazolin
   c. Ampicillin
   d. Isoniazid

142. Which of the following drugs can cause hearing loss?
   a. Cloxacillin
   b. Vancomycin
   c. Doxycycline
   d. Cefaclor

143. Which of the following drugs is used to treat herpes?
   a. Levofloxacin
   b. Valacyclovir
   c. Tobramycin
   d. Clarithromycin

144. Which of the following inhalers requires the patient rinse their mouth with water after using?
   a. Albuterol
   b. Serevent
   c. Combivent
   d. Flovent
145. Which of the following antihistamines is available over the counter?
   a. Loratadine
   b. Fexofenadine
   c. Cetirizine
   d. Hydroxyzine
146. An antitussive drug treats which of the following conditions?
   a. Depression
   b. Allergies
   c. Cough
   d. Tension headaches
147. Viagra is contraindicated with which of the following drugs?
   a. Benzodiazepines
   b. Loop diuretics
   c. Nitroglycerin
   d. Antidepressants
148. Coumadin is contraindicated with which of the following drugs?
   a. Percodan
   b. Percocet
   c. Amitriptyline
   d. Potassium chloride
149. Coumadin is in which pregnancy category?
   a. C
   b. A
   c. D
   d. X
150. What is the dosing frequency of Boniva?
   a. Once monthly
   b. Once daily
   c. Every morning
   d. Once weekly

Answers Practice Test #1

1. d	51. b	101. b
2. a	52. a	102. a
3. a	53. d	103. b
4. a	54. d	104. c
5. d	55. c	105. b
6. c	56. b	106. a
7. c	57. b	107. a
8. a	58. b	108. c
9. a	59. b	109. b
10. a	60. d	110. d
11. c	61. c	111. a
12. c	62. a	112. a
13. d	63. d	113. b
14. a	64. d	114. d
15. d	65. b	115. d
16. d	66. a	116. d
17. c	67. c	117. c
18. b	68. a	118. a
19. b	69. b	119. c
20. c	70. d	120. c
21. a	71. d	121. d
22. c	72. a	122. c
23. b	73. b	123. b
24. b	74. d	124. c
25. b	75. d	125. b
26. a	76. a	126. a
27. d	77. a	127. c
28. a	78. c	128. b
29. c	79. c	129. d
30. c	80. a	130. b
31. c	81. c	131. d
32. b	82. a	132. b
33. a	83. a	133. d
34. b	84. a	134. c
35. c	85. b	135. b
36. d	86. c	136. a
37. a	87. d	137. c
38. d	88. c	138. c
39. d	89. a	139. b
40. c	90. c	140. d
41. a	91. c	141. a
42. b	92. b	142. c
43. d	93. b	143. c
44. a	94. a	144. d
45. d	95. c	145. c
46. c	96. a	146. a
47. d	97. b	147. d
48. a	98. d	148. a
49. a	99. c	149. b
50. d	100. d	150. b

Solutions Practice Test #1

9. Rx   Carbamide Peroxide   6.5%
         Glycerin ad   60 mL
         Sig. Five drops in right ear.
How many grams of carbamide peroxide should be used to prepare this prescription?

$$\frac{6.5 \text{ g}}{100 \text{ mL}} = \frac{X}{60 \text{ mL}}$$

100 mL x X = 6.5 g x 60 mL
100 mL x X = 390 g x mL
$X = \frac{390 \text{ g x mL}}{100 \text{ mL}}$
X = 3.9 g

19. Rx   Keralac®   50%
Compound Benzoin Tincture ad 50 mL
     Sig. Apply to area of dry skin TID.
How many grams of Keralac® should be used to prepare this prescription?
$$\frac{50 \text{ g}}{100 \text{ mL}} = \frac{X}{50 \text{ mL}}$$
100 mL x X = 50 g x 50 mL
100 ml x X = 2500 g x mL
$X = \frac{2500 \text{ g x mL}}{100 \text{ mL}}$
X = 25 g

29. How many ml of 90% Dextrose should be mixed with water to make 1 liter of a 30% Dextrose solution?
     Remember water has a 0% concentration.
         1 liter = 1000 ml

```
90          30
      30    +
0           60
            90
```
For 90% solution: 30/90 x 1000 = 333 ml
For 0% solution: 60/90 x 1000 = 667 ml
     Check: 333 + 667 = 1000 ml

39. If an injection contains 1% (w/v) of diphenhydramine, calculate the number of milligrams of the drug in 50 mL of injection.

$$\frac{1 \text{ g}}{100 \text{ mL}} = \frac{X}{50 \text{ mL}}$$

X x 100 mL = 1 g x 50 mL
X x 100 mL = 50 g x mL
$X = \frac{50 \text{ g x mL}}{100 \text{ mL}}$
X = 0.5 g = 500 mg

49. How many ml of 70% ethanol should be mixed with water to make 1 liter of 50% ethanol solution?
         1 liter = 1000 ml

```
70          50
      50    +
0           20
            70
```

For 70% solution: 50/70 x 1000 = 714 ml
For 0% solution: 20/70 x 1000 = 286 ml
Check: 714 + 286 = 1000 ml

56. How many gallons are contained in 120 pints?
     8 pt = 1 gallon

$$\frac{8 \text{ pt}}{1 \text{ gal}} = \frac{120 \text{ pt}}{X}$$

120 pt x 1 gal = 8 pt x X

$$\frac{120 \text{ pt x gal}}{8 \text{ pt}} = \frac{8 \text{ pt x X}}{8 \text{ pt}}$$

15 gal = X

64. The physician orders 250 ml of Heparin to be infused over 15 hours. How many ml/hr should the IV pump be programmed for?

$$\frac{250 \text{ ml}}{15 \text{ hr}} = 16.7 \frac{\text{ml}}{\text{hr}}$$

71. What is 20% of 200?
20/100 = 0.2
0.2 x 200 = 40

80. In what proportion should 30% zinc oxide ointment be mixed with an ointment base to produce a 5% zinc oxide ointment?

30%   5 parts of 30% ointment
            5%
0%   25 parts of ointment base

Relative amounts: 5:25 or 1:5

88. How any milliliters of 70% alcohol should be mixed with a 10% alcohol solution to make 4500 ml of a 30% alcohol solution?

70%   20 parts of 70% alcohol
            30%
10%   40 parts of 10% alcohol
                       60
20 x 4500 = 1500 ml of 70%
60
40 x 4500 = 3000 ml of 10%
60

94. When using a 150 mg/ml solution, what volume would be needed to give a dose of 0.0750 gm?
$\frac{150mg}{1ml} = \frac{75mg}{X}$
(1ml)(75mg) = (150mg)(X)
$\frac{75 \text{ mg} \times ml}{150 \text{ mg}}$ = X
0.5ml = X

96. Label instructions for furosemide call for the addition of 9 mL of water to make 10 mL of reconstituted liquid such that each 5 mL contains 100 mg of furosemide. How much volume is occupied by the dry powder?

10 mL – 9 mL = 1 mL

97. From the previous question, what is the total amount of furosemide in the 10 mL product?
$\frac{5 \text{ mL}}{100 \text{ mg}} = \frac{10 \text{ mL}}{X}$

X x 5 mL = 100 mg x 10 mL
X x 5 mL = 1000 mg x mL
X = $\frac{1000 \text{ mg} \times \text{mL}}{5 \text{ mL}}$
X = 200 mg

98. Using the answer from the previous question, if a doctor orders a furosemide concentration of 75 mg/5 mL (rather than 100 mg/5 mL), how many milliliters of water should be added to the dry powder?
$\frac{200 \text{ mg}}{X} = \frac{75 \text{ mg}}{5 \text{ mL}}$

X x 75 mg = 200 mg x 5 mL
X x 75 mg = 1000 mg x mL
X = $\frac{1000 \text{ mg} \times \text{mL}}{75 \text{ mg}}$
X = 13.33 mL (volume of product that can be made with a concentration of 75 mg/ 5 mL)

13.33 mL – 1 mL (volume occupied by dry powder) = 12.33 mL

132. How much amoxicillin suspension 200 mg/5 ml is required for a dose of 250 mg?

$\frac{200 \text{ mg}}{5 \text{ mL}} = \frac{250 \text{ mg}}{X}$

200 mg x X = 250 mg x 5 mL
200 mg x X = 1250 mg x mL
X = $\frac{1250 \text{ mg} \times \text{mL}}{200 \text{ mg}}$
X = 6.25 mL = 1 ¼ tsp

137. An IV infusion order is received for Vancomycin 1000 mg in 1000 mL of NS, to be infused over 90 minutes. What will the flow rate be in mL/min?

$\frac{1000 \text{ mL}}{90 \text{ min}}$ = 11.11 mL/min

141. An administration set that delivers 15 gtt/mL is set up to infuse 500 mL D5W over a 12 hour period. What flow rate will be required to deliver the 500 mL?

$\frac{15 \text{ gtt}}{\text{mL}}$ x $\frac{500 \text{ mL}}{12 \text{ hr}}$ x $\frac{1 \text{ hr}}{60 \text{ min}}$ = 10.4 gtt/min

142. How many 500 mg doses are in a 100 mL bottle of 250 mg/ 5 mL Amoxicillin suspension?

100 mL x 250 mg/5 mL = 5000 mg
5000 mg/ 500 mg = 10 doses

143. What is the error percentage rate if 15 errors are detected in the preparation of 250 prescriptions?

15 errors/ 250 prescriptions = 0.06 x 100% = 6%

147. If the dosage of a medication is 90 mg/kg/day in two divided doses, what is the dose for a 40 lb child?

40 ~~lb~~ x 1 kg/2.2 ~~lb~~ = 18.18 kg
18.18 ~~kg~~ x 90 mg/~~kg~~/day = 1636.36 mg/day
1636.36 mg / 2 doses = 818.2 mg BID

150. How many grams would be administered when a drug order calls for 10 ml of a 20% solution?
10 ~~ml~~ x 20gm = 2gm
$\qquad$ 100~~ml~~

Answers Practice Test #2

1. c	51. a	101. c
2. c	52. a	102. d
3. d	53. d	103. d
4. b	54. b	104. d
5. d	55. b	105. a
6. b	56. b	106. b
7. b	57. b	107. d
8. c	58. a	108. a
9. d	59. d	109. a
10. a	60. d	110. b
11. d	61. b	111. c
12. b	62. b	112. c
13. c	63. a	113. c
14. a	64. c	114. b
15. d	65. c	115. d
16. b	66. d	116. c
17. b	67. c	117. c
18. c	68. d	118. a
19. c	69. b	119. a
20. b	70. a	120. a
21. b	71. b	121. c
22. d	72. a	122. I = a, II = b, III = c
23. a	73. b	123. b
24. b	74. c	124. a
25. a	75. c	125. c
26. c	76. b	126. c
27. b	77. b	127. a
28. b	78. b	128. b
29. b	79. c	129. b
30. d	80. a	130. d
31. a	81. c	131. b
32. c	82. c	132. c
33. c	83. b	133. a
34. d	84. b	134. c
35. d	85. d	135. b
36. a	86. a	136. b
37. a	87. a	137. d
38. b	88. a	138. c
39. c	89. a	139. d
40. d	90. b	140. a
41. b	91. b	141. a
42. a	92. d	142. c
43. c	93. c	143. d
44. c	94. d	144. a
45. c	95. a	145. a
46. d	96. c	146. b
47. b	97. c	147. c
48. a	98. a	148. b
49. d	99. a	149. a
50. d	100. c	150. c

Solutions Practice Test #2

10. Rx   Dipivefrin Hydrochloride 0.1%
         Solution   20 mL
         Sig. For the eye.
How many milligrams of dipivefrin hydrochloride should be used to prepare this prescription?

$$\frac{0.1\ g}{100\ mL} = \frac{X}{20\ mL}$$

0.1 g x 20 mL = X x 100 mL
2 g x mL = X x 100 mL

$$\frac{2\ g\ x\ mL}{100\ mL} = X$$

X = 0.02 g = 20 mg

15. If the dose of a medication is 80 mg/kg/day four times daily, how would a 195 lb patient be dosed?

195 lbs x $\frac{1 kg}{2.2 lbs}$ = 88.64kg x 80mg = 7091mg/day

20. A formula for a mouth rinse contains 1/25% (w/v) of potassium choride. How many grams of potassium chloride should be used in preparing 30 liters of the mouth rinse?

1/25% = 0.04%
100 mL = 0.1 L

$$\frac{0.04\ g}{0.1\ L} = \frac{X}{30\ L}$$

X x 0.1 L = 0.04 g x 30 L
X x 0.1 L = 1.2 g x L

$$X = \frac{1.2\ g\ x\ L}{0.1\ L}$$

X = 12 g

30. The intravenous dose of mannitol is 1.5 g/kg of body weight, administered as a 15 % (w/v) solution. How many milliliters of the solution should be administered to a 135 lb patient?

135 lb x $\frac{1\ kg}{2.2\ lb}$ = 61.36 kg

61.36 kg x 1.5 g/kg = 92.05 g

$$\frac{15\ g}{100\ mL} = \frac{92.05\ g}{X}$$

X x 15 g = 100 mL x 92.05 g
X x 15 g = 9205 mL x g

$$X = \frac{9205\ mL\ x\ g}{15\ g}$$

X = 613.67 mL or 614 mL

40. A pharmacist incorporates 10 gm of lidocaine into 150 gm of a 5% lidocaine ointment. Calculate the percentage (w/w) of lidocaine in the finished product.

$$\frac{X}{150\ gm} = \frac{5\ gm}{100\ gm}$$

(X)(100) = (150)(5)
X = 7.5 gm
7.5 gm x 10 gm = 17.5 gm

$$\frac{X}{100\ gm} = \frac{17.5\ gm}{160\ gm}$$

X x 160 gm = 100 gm x 17.5 gm
X x 160 gm = 1750 gm x gm

$$X = \frac{1750\ gm\ x\ gm}{160\ gm}$$

X = 10.9 gm

$$\frac{10.9\ gm}{100\ gm} = 10.9\ \%$$

51. How many grams of 35% lidocaine ointment should be mixed with petrolatum to prepare 3 lbs of 5% lidocaine ointment?

35%   5 parts 35% ointment
       5%   +
0%   30 parts of 0% petrolatum
                35 total parts

1 lbs = 454 gm
3 lbs = 3 x 454 gm = 1362 gm

$$\frac{5}{35} = \frac{X}{1362}$$

(5)(1362) = (35)(X)

$$\frac{6810}{35} = X$$

194.57 or 195 gm = X

59. How many grams of 5% (w/w) boric acid solution can be made from 1500 g of 50% (w/w) boric acid solution?

$$\frac{5\%}{50\%} = \frac{1500 \text{ g}}{X}$$

X x 5% = 1500 g x 50%
X x 5% = 75,000 g x %

$$X = \frac{75,000 \text{ g x } \cancel{\%}}{5\cancel{\%}}$$

X = 15,000 g

67. How much water should be mixed with 2500 ml of 75 % (v/v) alcohol to make 50 % (v/v) alcohol?

$$\frac{50 \%}{75 \%} = \frac{2500 \text{ mL}}{X}$$

X x 50 % = 2500 mL x 75 %
X x 50 % = 187,500 mL x %

$$X = \frac{187,500 \text{ mL x } \%}{50 \cancel{\%}}$$

X = 3750 mL

75. What is the percentage strength (v/v) of alcohol in a mixture of 2000 mL of 35% (v/v) alcohol, 750 mL of 55% (v/v) alcohol, and 750 mL of 65% (v/v) alcohol?

0.35	x	2000 mL	=	700 mL
0.55	x	750 mL	=	412.5 mL
0.65	x	750 mL	=	487.5 mL
Totals:		3500 mL		1600 mL

1600 mL /3500 mL = 0.457 x 100% = 45.7%

84. How many grams of 5% diphenhydramine cream should be mixed with 0.5% diphenhydramine cream to make 500 gm of 2% diphenhydramine cream?

5%   1.5 parts of 3% cream
        2%
0.5%   3   parts of 0.5% cream
             4.5 parts

$$\frac{1.5 \text{ parts}}{4.5 \text{ parts}} \text{ x 500 gm} = 167 \text{ gm of 5\% crm}$$

95. How many milliliters of a 60% (w/v) sucrose solution and how many milliliters of 10% (w/v) sucrose solution are required to prepare 5000 mL of a 20 % solution?

60%   10 parts of a 60% solution
        20%   +
10%   40 parts of a 10% solution
                    50

Relative amounts: 10:40 or 1:4, with a total of 5 parts

$$\frac{10 \text{ parts}}{50 \text{ parts}} \text{ x 5000 ml } = 1000 \text{ml of 60\% soln.}$$

$$\frac{40 \text{ parts}}{50 \text{ parts}} \text{ x 5000 ml } = 4000 \text{ ml of 10\% soln.}$$

104. The label of a dry powder for oral suspension states that when 98 mL of water are added to the powder, 150 mL of a suspension containing 300 mg of penicillin per 5 mL are prepared. How many milliliters of water should be used to prepare, in each 5 mL of product, the correct dose of penicillin for a 50 lb child based on the dose of 5 mg/kg of body weight?

Dose of penicillin:

$$\frac{5 \text{ mg}}{2.2 \text{ lb}} = \frac{X}{50 \text{ lb}}$$

X x 2.2 lb = 5 mg x 50 lb
X x 2.2 lb = 250 mg x lb

$$X = \frac{250 \text{ mg x } \cancel{\text{lb}}}{2.2 \cancel{\text{lb}}}$$

X = 113.6 mg

The amount of penicillin in the container:

$$\frac{300 \text{ mg}}{5 \text{ mL}} = \frac{X}{150 \text{ mL}}$$

X x 5 mL = 300 mg x 150 mL
X x 5 mL = 45,000 mg x mL

$$X = \frac{45,000 \text{ mg x } \cancel{\text{mL}}}{5 \cancel{\text{mL}}}$$

X = 9000 mg

The amount of product that can be made from 9000 mg of drug such that each 5 mL contains 113.6 mg of drug:

$$\frac{113.6 \text{ mg}}{5 \text{ mL}} = \frac{9000 \text{ mg}}{X}$$

X x 113.6 mg = 5 mL x 9000 mg
X x 113.6 mg = 45,000 mg x mL

$$X = \frac{45,000 \cancel{\text{mg}} \text{ x mL}}{113.6 \cancel{\text{mg}}}$$

X = 396.13 mL

Because the volume of powder occupies 52 mL (150 mL – 98 mL), the amount of water to add is determined by:

$$396.13 \text{ mL} – 52 \text{ mL} = 344.13 \text{ mL}$$

138. What amount of 100% lanolin ointment must be diluted with white petrolatum to fill an order for 1/2 pound of 15% lanolin ointment? [Remember 1 lb = 454 g]

100%   15 parts 100% lanolin oint
          15%
0%   85 parts white petrolatum
                        100

Relative amounts: 15:85 or 3:17, with a total of 20 parts

15 parts x 227 gm = **34.05 gm of 100% lanolin**
100 parts
85 parts x 227 gm = 192.95 gm of petrolatum
100 parts

140. You have an order for a solution of 2% dextrose in NS to be given in a 5- hour IV infusion. The Pharmacy has a 500 ml IV bag of saline and a 40% dextrose solution in stock. What volume of the 40% solution should be added to the IV bag?

40%   2 parts 40%
          2%   +
0%   38 parts NS
                       40

2 parts   x 500ml = 25 ml of 40% soln.
40 parts

142. A patient is taking three 600 mg capsules of lithium each day. How much lithium would the patient take in 30 days?

3 x 600 mg = 1800 mg x 30 days = 54,000 mg

143. An IV infustion order is received for piperacillin-tazobactam (Zosyn) 3.375 g in 500 mL of NS to be infused at 113 mg/min. What will the flow rate be in mL/hr?

$$\frac{500 \text{ mL}}{3375 \text{ mg}} \times \frac{113 \text{ mg}}{\text{min}} \times \frac{60 \text{ min}}{\text{hr}} = 1004.4 \text{ mL/hr}$$

144. An IV infusion order is received for furosemide (Lasix) 40 mg in 500 mL of NS, to be infused at 75 mL/hr. What amount of furosemide will the patient receive per hour?

$$\frac{75 \text{ mL}}{\text{hr}} \times \frac{40 \text{ mg}}{500 \text{ mL}} = 6 \text{ mg/hr}$$

146. A 500 ml bag of 0.25%NS runs at 60 gtt/min with an infusion delivering 10 gtt/ml. How long will the infusion go?

$$500 \text{ mL} \times \frac{10 \text{ gtts}}{\text{mL}} \times \frac{\text{min}}{60 \text{ gtts}} \times \frac{1 \text{ hr}}{60 \text{ mins}} = 1.39 \text{ hr}$$

149. If 20 gallons of distilled water cost $45.25, how much will 5 gallons cost?

$$\frac{20 \text{ gallons}}{\$45.25} = \frac{5 \text{ gallons}}{X}$$

20 gallons x X = 5 gallons x $45.25
20 gallons x X = $226.25 x gallons

$$X = \frac{\$226.25 \text{ x gallons}}{20 \text{ gallons}}$$
X = $11.31

150. An order of amoxicillin 250 mg BID for 10 days. If a 100 mg/5 mL suspension is used, the volume of each dose will be?

250 mg x 5 mL/ 100 mg = 12.5 mL

Answers Practice Test #3

1. c	51. d	101. d
2. c	52. c	102. c
3. c	53. d	103. d
4. c	54. d	104. b
5. c	55. c	105. a
6. a	56. d	106. b
7. c	57. c	107. a
8. d	58. d	108. d
9. c	59. a	109. d
10. a	60. a	110. a
11. b	61. c	111. d
12. c	62. a	112. b
13. b	63. b	113. d
14. b	64. b	114. a
15. d	65. b	115. a
16. a	66. c	116. a
17. c	67. c	117. b
18. b	68. b	118. c
19. b	69. b	119. e
20. d	70. d	120. a
21. a	71. b	121. d
22. d	72. c	122. a
23. d	73. b	123. c
24. d	74. a	124. c
25. b	75. d	125. a
26. c	76. c	126. d
27. c	77. a	127. b
28. a	78. d	128. a
29. c	79. b	129. c
30. a	80. a	130. b
31. b	81. b	131. c
32. b	82. b	132. b
33. c	83. a	133. a
34. b	84. d	134. c
35. d	85. b	135. d
36. d	86. c	136. d
37. a	87. d	137. b
38. c	88. c	138. d
39. d	89. a	139. c
40. a	90. b	140. b
41. b	91. b	141. d
42. b	92. b	142. b
43. c	93. b	143. b
44. c	94. d	144. d
45. c	95. c	145. a
46. b	96. b	146. c
47. b	97. c	147. c
48. d	98. c	148. a
49. a	99. d	149. d
50. b	100. b	150. a

Solutions Practice Test #3

6. If 0.025 gm thyroid extract contains 50 mcg of levothyroxine, how much levothyroxine is contained in 2.5 mg of thyroid extract?

$$\frac{25 \text{ mg thyroid ext}}{50 \text{ mcg l-thyroxine}} = \frac{2.5 \text{ mg thyroid ext}}{X}$$

25mg thyroid x X = 2.5mg thyroid x 50 mcg l-thyroxine

25mg thyroid x X = 125mg thyroid x mcg l-thyroxine

$$X = \frac{125 \text{ mg thyroid} \times \text{mcg l-thyroxine}}{25 \text{ mg thyroid}}$$

X = 5 mcg l-thyroxine

7. A pharmacy technician wants to add 75 mg of a particular drug to 100 mL of NS. The drug solution is supplied in a 2% concentration. What is the volume of the 2% concentration required to supply 75 mg of the drug?

$$\frac{2 \text{ grams}}{100 \text{ mL}} = \frac{0.075 \text{ grams}}{X}$$

2 grams x X = 100 mL x 0.075 grams
2 grams x X = 7.5 mL x grams

$$X = \frac{7.5 \text{ mL} \times \text{grams}}{2 \text{ grams}}$$

X = 3.75 mL

8. A 66-lb child is given a prescription for Amoxicillin. The recommended child dose is 25mg/kg/day in two doses. What is the correct dose to be given?

$$66 \text{ lbs} \times \frac{1 \text{ kg}}{2.2 \text{ lbs}} = 30 \text{ kg}$$

$$\frac{25 \text{ mg}}{\text{kg}} \times 30 \text{ kg} = 750 \text{mg per day}$$

750mg per day / 2 doses = 375mg

14. A pharmacy fills an order for 30 Cipro tablets containing 0.250 g of ciprofloxacin each. How much ciprofloxacin is dispensed?

30 x 250mg = 7500 mg

15. How much ciprofloxacin suspension 250 mg/5 mL would be needed to fill a prescription for ciprofloxacin 500 mg PO q12h for 10 days?

500 mg x 2 x 10 days = 10,000 mg
10,000 mg x 5 mL/250 mg = 200 mL

16. A liquid contains 0.5 mg/mL of a substance. How much of the substance will 4.2 L contain?

4200 mL x 0.5 mg/mL = 2100 mg

17. A prescription order specifies potassium chloride 20 mEq po BID. What volume of KCl solution containing 20 mEq/15 mL will be required to deliver a single dose?

20 mEq x 15 mL/20 mEq = 15 mL

26. If 200 tablets contain 400 mg of a substance, how many grains would 600 tablets contain?

$$\frac{200 \text{ tablets}}{400 \text{ mg}} = \frac{600 \text{ tablets}}{X}$$

200 tablets x X = 600 tablets x 400 mg
200 tablets x X = 240,000 tablets x mg

$$X = \frac{240,000 \text{ tablets} \times \text{mg}}{200 \text{ tablets}}$$

X = 1200 mg

1200 mg x 1 grain/65 mg = 18.5 grains

27. The metric equivalent of a 5 grain dose of Amoxil is:

5 grain x 65 mg/grain = 325 mg

28. If 2 kg of a cream contains 500 g of triamcinolone, what is the percentage strength of the cream?

$$\frac{X\%}{100 \text{ g}} = \frac{500 \text{ g}}{2000 \text{ g}}$$

X x 2000g = 100g x 500g
X x 2000g = 50,000 g x g

$$X = \frac{50,000 \text{ g} \times \text{g}}{2000 \text{ g}}$$

X = 25 g or 25%

191

31. What volume of Pepto Bismol would be dispensed to administer a dose of 2 oz?

2 ~~oz~~ x 30 mL/ ~~oz~~ = 60 mL

32. A cash discount of $250 on a pharmacy invoice for $7700 represents a percentage cash discount of:

$250/ $7700 = 0.0325 x 100% = 3.25%

33. A 40 mL dose of a mixture prescribed for pain relief contains 30 mg codeine, 325 mg acetaminophen, 10 mL grape syrup q.s. with water. How many 60 mg codeine tables are needed to prepare 480 mL of this solution?

$$\frac{40 \text{ mL}}{30 \text{ mg}} = \frac{480 \text{ mL}}{X}$$

40 mL x X = 480 mL x 30 mg
40 mL x X = 14,400 mL x mg
$$X = \frac{14,400 \text{ mL} \times \text{mg}}{40 \text{ mL}}$$
X = 360 mg
360 ~~mg~~ x 1 tablet/ 60 ~~mg~~ = 6 tablets

47. A patient is to be administered a drug that has a recommended dosage of 2 mg/kg of body weight. The patient is a child weighing 40 lbs. The amount of the drug the patient is to receive is:

40 ~~lbs~~ x kg/ 2.2 ~~lbs~~ = 18.18 kg
18.18 ~~kg~~ x 2 mg/ ~~kg~~ = 36.4 mg

48. How much nystatin must be added to triamcinolone cream to dispense an order for 60 g of triamcinolone cream with 2% nystatin?

$$\frac{2 \text{ g}}{100 \text{ g}} = \frac{X}{60 \text{ g}}$$

100 g x X = 2 g x 60 g
100 g x X = 120 g x g
$$X = \frac{120 \text{ g} \times \text{g}}{100 \text{ g}}$$
X = 1.2 g or 1200 mg

49. A prescription requires a 50 mg dose of Diazepam IV, and the pharmacy only stocks vials of 10 mg/mL. What volume of this solution will be required to dispense the correct dose?

50 ~~mg~~ x mL/10 ~~mg~~ = 5 mL

50. How many 875 mg amoxicillin tablets are required to prepare 1000 mL of a 250 mg/ 5 mL concentration?

1000 ~~mL~~ x 250 mg/ 5 ~~mL~~ = 50,000 mg
50,000 mg x 1 tablet/ 875 mg = 57.14 tablet or 58 tablets

60. A Heparin drip is given at a concentration of 25 units/mL and dosed at 1000 units/hr. How many mL/hr would be given to the patient?

1000 ~~units~~/hr x mL/ 25 ~~units~~ = 40 mL/hr

61. How many grams of Dextrose are contained in a 5 mL solution of Dextrose 25%?

$$\frac{25 \text{ g}}{100 \text{ mL}} = \frac{X}{5 \text{ mL}}$$

100 mL x X = 25 g x 5 mL
100 mL x X = 125 g x mL
$$X = \frac{125 \text{ g} \times \text{mL}}{100 \text{ mL}}$$
X = 1.25 g

62. What volume of 3 mEq/mL NaCl injection must be added to a TPN solution to deliver 40 mEq of NaCl?

40 ~~mEq~~ x mL/ 3 ~~mEq~~ = 13.33 mL

73. What daily dose of a drug prescribes at 30 mg/kg/day would be administered to a patient weighing 75 kg?

75 ~~kg~~ x 30 mg/ ~~kg~~ /day = 2250 mg/day

74. What dosage will be delivered by the infusion of 500 mL of an IV solution containing 0.5 mg/mL of a medication?

500 ~~mL~~ x 0.5 mg/ ~~mL~~ = 250 mg

75. A child is to receive an amoxicillin dosage of 40 mg/kg/day in equally divided doses every 8 hours. Which of the following manufacturer's product sizes should be used to reconstitute a 10 day supply of suspension for a 80 lb child if the label reads 400 mg/5 mL?

80 lbs x kg/2.2 lbs = 36.4 kg
36.4 ~~kg~~ x 40 mg/~~kg~~ /day = 1454.5 mg/day
1454.5 mg/day x 10 days = 14545 mg
14545 mg x 5 mL/400 mg = 181.8 mL

Use a 200 mL bottle.

87. 112 ml is equivalent to how many fluid ounces?

1 oz = 30 ml

$$\frac{1\ oz}{30\ ml} = \frac{X}{112\ ml}$$

112 ml x 1 oz = 30 ml x X

$$\frac{112\ \cancel{ml}\ x\ oz}{30\ \cancel{ml}} = \frac{30\ \cancel{ml}\ x\ X}{30\ \cancel{ml}}$$

3.73 oz = X

88. 150 grams is equivalent to how many mg?

Multiply by 1000 or move to the right three spaces
$$150\ \cancel{g}\ x\ \frac{1000\ mg}{1\ \cancel{g}} = 150,000\ mg$$

98. How much Ceclor 250 mg per 2.5 ml suspension should be dispensed for a 350 mg dose?

$$\frac{250\ mg}{2.5\ ml} = \frac{350\ mg}{X}$$

350 mg x 2.5 ml = 250 mg x X

875 mg x ml = 250 mg x X

$$\frac{875\ \cancel{mg}\ x\ ml}{250\ \cancel{mg}} = X$$

3.5 ml = X

99. What volume of a 100 mg/ml injectable should be drawn up for 120 mg dose?

$$\frac{100\ mg}{1\ ml} = \frac{120\ mg}{X}$$

1ml x 120 mg = 100 mg x X

120 ml x mg = 100 mg x X

$$\frac{120\ ml\ x\ \cancel{mg}}{100\ \cancel{mg}} = X$$

1.2 ml = X

107. Nitrostat 1/400 grains is equivalent to how many milligrams?

$$\frac{1}{400} = 0.0025\ gr$$

$$\frac{1\ gr}{60\ mg} = \frac{0.0025\ gr}{X}$$

60 mg x 0.0025 gr = 1 gr x X

$$\frac{0.15\ mg\ x\ \cancel{gr}}{1\ \cancel{gr}} = \frac{1\ \cancel{gr}\ x\ X}{1\ \cancel{gr}}$$

0.15 mg = X

108. How many 100 mg doses are contained in 15 g of Cephalexin?

Convert 15 g to mg
Multiply 15 g x 1000 = 15000 mg
$$\frac{15000}{100} = 150\ doses$$

109. A 600 tablet bottle of ferrous sulfate cost $ 105.00. What would be the cost of 150 tablets?

$$\frac{105}{600} = \frac{X}{150}$$
105 x 150 = 600 x X
15750 = 600 x X
$$\frac{15750}{600} = X$$
$26.25 = X

110. A 350 tablet bottle of ferrous sulfate cost $ 9.50. What would be the cost of 35 tablets?

$$\frac{9.50}{350} = \frac{X}{35}$$

9.50 x 35 = 350 x X
332.5 = 350 x X

$$\frac{332.5}{350} = X$$
$0.95 = X

117. The cost of 1000 tablets of ibuprofen 200 mg is $ 50.99. If your pharmacy markups the cost by 10%, what would be the retail charge for 50 tablets?

$50.99 x 0.10 = $5.10

$50.99 + $5.10 = $56.09

$\dfrac{\$56.09}{1000} = \dfrac{X}{50}$

$56.09 x 50 = 1000 x X

$2804.50 = 1000 x X

$\dfrac{\$2804.50}{1000} = X$

$2.80 = X

127. The AWP for a drug $ 65.99 with a 10% discount from the wholesaler. What would be the cost of this drug?

$\dfrac{10}{100} = 0.10$

$65.99 x 0.10 = $6.60

$65.99 - $6.60 = $59.39

128. The AWP for a drug $ 26.99 with a 5% discount from the wholesaler. What would be the cost of this drug?

$\dfrac{5}{100} = 0.05$

$26.99 x 0.05 = $1.35

$26.99 - $1.35 = $25.64

129. How many grams of a 2% hydrocortisone cream can be made from 350 grams of 4% cream?

S1 4/100 = 0.04

S2 2/100 = 0.02

Q1 = 350g

Q2 = X

0.04 x 350g = 0.02 x X

14 = 0.02 x X

14/0.02 = X

700 g = X

130. How much of 50% ethanol must be mixed with 25% ethanol to make 1 pint of 35% ethanol solution?

1 pint = 480 ml

```
50              10
        35     +
25              15
                25
```

For 50 % solution: 10/25 x 480 = 192 ml

For 25 % solution: 15/25 x 480 = 288 ml

Check: 192 + 288 + 480 ml

131. If a dose of Cephalexin is 34 mg/kg/day and the patient weights 54 lbs. How many milligrams will be given daily?

1 kg = 2.2 lbs

54 ~~lbs~~ x $\dfrac{1 \text{ kg}}{2.2 \text{lbs}}$ = 24.5 kg

24.5~~kg~~ x $\dfrac{34 \text{mg}}{\text{kg}}$ = 833 mg per day

137. Determine the flow rate of an IV if 125 ml of drug is to be infused over 2 hours. The administration set delivers 60 gtts/ml.

2 hours = 120 minutes

$\dfrac{125 \text{ ml}}{120 \text{ min}}$ x $\dfrac{60 \text{gtts}}{\text{ml}}$ = X

$\dfrac{7500 \text{ } \bcancel{ml} \text{ x gtts}}{120 \text{ min x } \bcancel{ml}}$ = X

$\dfrac{63 \text{ gtts}}{\text{min}}$ = X

138. Determine the flow rate of an IVPB containing 150 ml of gentamycin. The solution is to be infused over a 1 hour period and the administration set is calibrated to deliver 10 drops per ml.

$\dfrac{150 \text{ml}}{60 \text{min}}$ x $\dfrac{10 \text{gtts}}{\text{ml}}$ = X

$\dfrac{1500 \text{ } \bcancel{ml} \text{ x gtts}}{60 \text{ min x } \bcancel{ml}}$ = X

$\dfrac{25 \text{ gtts}}{\text{min}}$ = X

NOTES

CPSIA information can be obtained at www.ICGtesting.com
Printed in the USA
LVOW100625300513

336127LV00001B/2/A